PENGUIN BOOKS

THE RUNNER'S TRAINING DIARY

BOB GLOVER is founder and president of Robert H. Glover and Associates, Inc., a sports and fitness consulting firm. Since he founded the program in 1978, Glover has directed the running classes for the 32,000-member New York Road Runners Club. More than 3,000 students participate each year in these classes at the beginner runner through advanced competitive levels. Glover also directs the training clinics for the New York City Marathon. His Official New York City Marathon Training Program is followed annually by thousands of runners. Each year since its founding in 1990, Glover has directed more than 1,000 boys and girls aged six to thirteen in the City-Sports-For-Kids track and field program sponsored by the New York Road Runners Club and the Asphalt Green. A high school (Dansville, New York) county champion at two miles and a three-time gold medalist at the Hue Sports Festival during the Vietnam War, he has competed for more than thirty-five years at distances ranging from the quarter-mile to the 50-mile ultramarathon, and has completed more than 30 marathons. He now places frequently in local races as a masters runner (age 50-plus division), competing for the Westchester Track Club. Glover has coached three women athletes to U.S. top-10 rankings in the marathon event, and has coached his running teams to several national titles at a variety of distances in both the open and masters categories. He has more than twenty-five years' experience coaching all levels of runners. More than fifty thousand runners have participated in his classes, and nearly a million runners have followed his training program in his books since *The Runner's Handbook* was first published and became an immediate national bestseller in 1978. He and his wife, Shelly-lynn, live in Sleepy Hollow, New York, where they love to run together along wooded trails. They often win awards in couples races.

SHELLY-LYNN FLORENCE GLOVER is an exercise physiologist with a master's degree from Columbia University as well as certification as a fitness professional from the American Council on Exercise and Marymount Manhattan College. She has an undergraduate degree in journalism. As a researcher, she has been active in several studies involving runners. Her work involving "critical velocity" as a means of predicting marathon times was accepted for publication and was presented at the 1995 American College of Sports Medicine Conference in Minneapolis. She competed for her high school (Canisteo, New York) track team, was co-captain of the soccer team, and was a member of her college's first women's cross-country team. As a veteran of more than twenty years of racing, she competes for the Westchester Track Club and frequently wins awards in local races ranging in distance from 5K to the marathon. She is founder and president of Great Strides, which specializes in personalized training programs. She also founded and coaches Mercury Masters, a women's running team for athletes who are over the age of fifty, and City Striders, a running team for boys and girls. As program director for Glover and Associates, she coaches with the New York Road Runners Club's City-Sports-For-Kids youth track program and the NYRRC's adult running classes.

IN MEMORY
Dr. Murray Weisenfeld treated thousands of runners in over
forty years of service as a podiatrist in New York City. He wrote the
popular *Runner's Repair Manual* and co-authored, with me,
The Injured Runner's Training Handbook. Murray was my advisor,
my personal sports doctor, and—most important—my good friend.
—Bob Glover

ALSO BY BOB GLOVER AND SHELLY-LYNN FLORENCE GLOVER
The Runner's Handbook
The Competitive Runner's Handbook

ALSO BY BOB GLOVER
The Injured Runner's Training Handbook
The Family Fitness Handbook

The Runner's
Training Diary

FOR
FITNESS
RUNNERS
AND
COMPETITIVE
RACERS

**Bob Glover and
Shelly-lynn Florence Glover**

 PENGUIN BOOKS

PENGUIN BOOKS
Published by the Penguin Group
Penguin Books USA Inc., 375 Hudson Street,
New York, New York 10014, U.S.A.
Penguin Books Ltd, 27 Wrights Lane,
London W8 5TZ, England
Penguin Books Australia Ltd, Ringwood,
Victoria, Australia
Penguin Books Canada Ltd, 10 Alcorn Avenue,
Toronto, Ontario, Canada M4V 3B2
Penguin Books (N.Z.) Ltd, 182–190 Wairau Road,
Auckland 10, New Zealand

Penguin Books Ltd, Registered Offices:
Harmondsworth, Middlesex, England

First published in Penguin Books 1997

10   9   8   7   6

A Note to the Reader
The ideas, procedures, and suggestions contained in this book are not intended to substitute for medical or other professional advice applicable to specific individuals. As with any activity program, yours should be prepared in consultation with a physician or other competent professional.

LIBRARY OF CONGRESS CATALOGING IN PUBLICATION DATA
Glover, Bob.
        The runner's training diary: for fitness runners and competitive racers/Bob Glover and Shelly-lynn Florence Glover.
            p.   cm.
        "Featuring the official New York City Marathon training program."
        ISBN 0 14 04.6991 5
        1. Marathon running—Training.   2. Marathon running.   I. Glover, Shelly-lynn Florence.
II. Title.
        GV1065.17.T73G56   1997
        796.42'52—dc21   96-49050

Printed in the United States of America
Set in Adobe Garamond
Designed by Jessica Shatan

CONTENTS

PART IV: THE MARATHON

PART V: REFERENCE CHARTS

Training Year: _____

GOALS FOR THE YEAR

INTRODUCTION

This book is unique and valuable for several reasons. First, it includes plenty of blank diary pages and charts that you fill in yourself. Thus you become the author of your own personal book of running. Second, it contains many training and reference charts from the best-selling *Runner's Handbook* and *The Competitive Runner's Handbook* to help guide you with your running.

Your diary is divided into five sections:

1. The *diary* consists of pages and charts to record all the key aspects of daily runs.

2. The *racing* section includes several charts to help plan, record, and analyze races.

3. The *training* section features sample training schedules for the Beginner Runner, Advanced Beginner Runner, Intermediate Runner, Novice Competitor, Basic Competitor, Competitor, and Advanced Competitor. These are the official training programs for the New York Road Runners Club running classes. These schedules and charts provide the outline for the training program you can write daily in your diary. For more comprehensive training guidelines, refer to *The Runner's Handbook* (for Beginner and Intermediate Runners) and *The Competitive Runner's Handbook*.

4. The *marathon* section features the official training schedule and guidelines for the New York City Marathon. *The Competitive Runner's Handbook* includes several chapters detailing how to train for and race the marathon distance—whether you are a novice or veteran marathoner.

5. The *reference* section includes several handy charts that will be useful to runners of all levels.

PART I

The Training Diary

Why Keep a Training Diary?

Since 1973 I have faithfully maintained a training diary, and Shelly-lynn's been keeping one since 1978. My diary has been there with me during all my ups and downs. I brag to it about significant mileage weeks, good workouts and races. I complain to it about my fatigue, poor runs and races, as well as injuries and illnesses. I pull my good friend off the shelf every day and talk to it. I record at least the basics: how far I ran, the pace of the run, and the course. By recording and graphing weekly mileage, I am able to use my diary to help coach me to keep on a consistent, progressive schedule. My diary-coach also contains all the essentials about my speed training and races so I can measure improvement.

I strongly recommend you keep a training diary, too. It will become a record of fitness and competition over a period of days, weeks, months, and years. A diary is essential to understanding what does and doesn't work in your running. You can study the past to succeed in the future. It will document your progress as a runner. You'll refer to it regularly for guidance. How did I train for my best races? How many long runs did I do going into my previous marathons? What was my running weight when I was racing well two years ago? What training errors contributed to my shin splints three months ago? What shoes did I wear in my previous marathon? Your training diary will have the answers to all these questions as well as a summary of your running highlights (and low points).

The training diary kept over the years also offers the opportunity to look back and reflect upon a memorable running career. I find that an old training diary is enjoyable reading. Reviewing my past successes as a competitive runner in the "good ol' days" makes me feel more assured of my running as a masters competitor.

Your diary gives you the opportunity to plan and analyze your training as a self-coached runner. It can inspire you to greatness! But remember that your diary—like any good coach or running partner—should be a motivator, not an overbearing stress. It should act like your conscience, urging you to get out the door to keep on schedule, but it should also be a voice of caution, reminding you of past training errors.

A diary can tell you in retrospect what you have done right or wrong. You can look back at the weeks preceding an injury or poor racing performance and find the telltale entries. More positively, you can review what training preceded good performances and build on this knowledge in the future.

The late Dr. George Sheehan emphasized that all runners "are an experiment of one." You learn what works best for you by trial and error. By experimenting with your running and keeping a detailed diary, you can write a personalized training book that is more valuable than any other book you could buy. Have fun writing your book of running!

How to Use Your Training Diary

Be consistent in keeping your diary. Fill information in after each workout, before you forget details. I set my diary on my desk when I return from my run and then fill it in after taking my shower. It is easier to reach weekly mileage goals if you record runs daily. A diary keeps you honest. Nobody likes to see too many unplanned zeros—*in writing*. But don't become a slave to recording mileage. Remember, fitness and performance are the goals, not accumulating mileage in your diary. By keeping a diary, you can make sure you do enough, but not too much, running to meet your goals.

Your daily and weekly records should at least include the basics: date, course, distance, running time, and pace. It may be useful to record even more information than I suggest. Most will choose to write less. You decide what is most valuable. Some runners opt to include personal entries unrelated to running. Wouldn't it be fun to browse through the diaries of some running friends!

THE WEEKLY TRAINING DIARY

The following 52 Week-by-Week Training Diary includes plenty of space to record the details of your running life. Here are some suggestions of what to log.

Day and Date

Record the day and date of each run in the designated box. I also note the training week at the top of each left-hand page for quick reference when I'm flipping through the pages. You can start with any day that you choose. I prefer Mondays. It is the beginning of the work or school week for most of us. So it just seems logical to start your running week then too. If you end a training week with a full weekend, you have more flexibility to use both Saturday and Sunday to meet mileage goals. Further, most races are held on Sunday. It is better to plan your week in your diary going into a race than starting with a race. This will enable you to do a better job with your prerace tapering and mental preparation.

I also write the training year on the outside cover of my diaries. Then I store them on a shelf in order, starting with 1973.

Running Time

Record the total time of your run. This is where your runner's watch with the chronograph mode comes in handy. I pause my watch if I'm stopping for more than a few seconds for whatever reason. Some runners prefer tracking only total minutes instead of mileage in their diary and keep daily and weekly time totals rather than mileage. But most of us will keep track of both the distance and time of each run and just track weekly mileage totals. Caution: It is easy to become obsessed with trying to run faster times over your courses. This is racing, not training, and will lead to injury or burnout. Keep yourself from running too hard to impress your diary.

Running Pace

Many runners are overly concerned about pace. Few of us have the luxury of exactly measured courses, so the actual pace we run is only an estimate anyway. You can approximate pace per mile by perceived exertion. None of my courses up and down wooded trails are accurately measured. My eight-miler, for example, is a loop course that usually takes me about 64 minutes while running at what feels like my normal eight-minute-per-mile training pace. At this pace my training heart rate is about 130 beats per minute, and I can converse comfortably. I'll record "approx. 8" in my diary in the pace column.

At times I'll run a measured course (a known trail or the high school track) to get a feel for my pace per mile. Another method to determine whether I'm running at about my normal training pace (or faster or slower) over my unmeasured courses is to note my running time at various checkpoints. I usually hit the underpass, for example, at about 13 minutes on my runs and that usually correlates to an eight-minute-per-mile pace. At least occasionally you may wish to accurately measure the time and distance of your run so that you can monitor your fitness.

But remember to note the weather and the course, because heat, humidity, winds, hills, and so on will slow the pace for a given effort.

Except for speed training and racing, your training pace should keep you within a training heart rate range of about 70 percent to 80 percent of your maximum heart rate. Refer to the Training Heart Rate Guide on page 157. At these paces, you should be able to converse in comfort. For most experienced competitors, this pace will translate to about one to two minutes per mile slower than your present 10K race pace. Refer to the Training Pace Guide on page 158.

Mileage

Most runners are mileage maniacs. We train so many miles per week, per month, per year. Mileage is the backbone of every runner's program. Too little and you fade before the finish line; too much and you don't make it to the starting line healthy.

As with training pace, you don't have to be obsessed with accurate measurements. You can just run, keeping track of time. When finished, estimate mileage based on the pace per mile you think you ran. I record to the nearest half mile, or use a plus or minus sign. For example, "8+" means that my run was probably more than 8 miles but not 8½ miles.

This diary also includes a daily mileage-to-date column. This tally makes it easier to keep on target for weekly goals. In your weekly summary section record total mileage for the week and the year to date.

Use the Week-by-Week Mileage Chart (page 116) to monitor the overall flow of mileage. I highlight my week-by-week entries by various mileage goals. For example, I asterisk a 60-mile week and circle a 70-mile week. Use the space for comments to record factors that influenced that week of running: a work project, family priorities, injury or illness, a race, heavy snow, and so on. I'll even congratulate myself with a comment such as "WOW" after moving up to a new mileage level.

The Training Mileage Graph (page 118) can be used to monitor your consistency (or lack of). It is valuable to watch the pattern of your own personal graph. The mileage guides on pages 156 and 165 will help you plan your weekly mileage for races of 5K to the marathon.

Weight

Each weigh-in should be without clothes and conducted at the same time of day. Competitive runners will improve performance the closer they come to the weight they can maintain and still be strong and healthy. Refer to the Performance Weight Chart for Runners on page 178. A morning weight loss of more than two pounds may indicate dehydration, so take this as a warning sign to rehydrate.

Heart Rate

Two types of heart rate are valuable to record. First, your resting heart rate is a good indicator of fitness level and recovery from hard training. A few times per week take your resting heart rate before getting out of bed in the morning. As you become fitter, your resting heart rate will lower. If your resting heart rate is 5 to 10 (or more) beats higher than normal, it may be a sign that you haven't yet recovered fully from training or your body is fighting off an illness. I note my resting heart rate in my diary as such, "50R." Check your heart rate during training periodically to see whether you are staying within your training heart rate range (see chart on page 157). Measuring your effort with a heart rate monitor is a good way to keep from running too hard. The monitor will help you concentrate on running at a steady effort rather than racing your watch. I wear my heart rate monitor a few times each week and note in my diary my average heart rate for the run, such as "128T." As you get in better shape, you will be able to run the same course, at the same pace, with a lower training heart rate.

Course

Note here where you ran. I describe my favorite courses (detailing the various landmarks so that I don't forget the exact route for later runs) on the chart on page 122 and then just refer to the name I give my course in the daily entry. For example, I'll enter "Lake 7" for my seven-mile course that loops Swan Lake. If I run a course that isn't one of my regular routes, then I'll detail it in my daily entry. Note the terrain: hilly, icy, dirt trails, and so on. By noting the exact course you ran, you can monitor how you feel running a given pace over the same route compared with previous (or future) runs.

Comments

This diary provides plenty of space to record valuable factors related to your running. Here are some examples: time of day, weather, sleep patterns, illness, running partners, menstrual cycle, details of a speed workout or race, stretching, weight training, cross-training. (For more information on stretching, weight training, and cross-training, see *The*

Runner's Handbook or *The Competitive Runner's Handbook*.) Check the boxes indicating a weight training or stretching session. Note in the cross-training entry any running equivalent. Determine this by how many miles you would have run during the time you cross-trained. For example, a 30-minute bike ride within your training heart rate range is equal to a four-mile run if you normally train at 7½ minutes per mile. You can even track the mileage on your shoes, so that after 300 to 500 miles you'll know it's time to replace them. Make note of your body's warning signs and management of injury. The Injury Chart on page 124 can be used to help you learn from your injuries.

You may also choose to comment on how you felt during your runs. Words like sluggish, stiff, sore, and heavy can describe a poor or fair run. And great, peppy, awesome, and terrific help describe a good or excellent workout. You may wish to add phrases such as "started too fast," "faded in the heat," or "still tired from long run" to further detail your experience. You may even wish to grade your runs. For example, you may score A for an excellent run, B for a good one, C for an average run, D for a fair one, and F for a run you'd like to forget. Be sure to note why you felt you had a bad run and what the symptoms were. Don't expect to have a great run every time you go out. Shelly-lynn tells her clients that for every five runs, most runners can expect to have one excellent run and one that is fair or worse. The other three will be average.

Weekly Summary

Record here your total mileage (or minutes) for the week and your total for the year to date. You may choose to record your average weekly mileage to date. Also note your longest run for the week. List your total number of runs for the week: Remember the goal is to run at least three times, preferably five or six times per week. Also note the total number of speed training, cross-training, weight training, and stretching workouts, to help you review your overall fitness program.

Use the blank space to write in the highlights and low points of your week's running. Examples: "Fourth straight week at 40 miles and I'm feeling stronger," "Weight below 165 for first time in 5 years," "Heat wave all week caused me to cut back," "Swam and biked an equivalent of 10 miles of running," "Allergies starting to act up again," "Took two days off to nurse sore Achilles." This section can serve as a quick progress check as you flip through the pages and review trends in your training.

SAMPLE TRAINING DIARY

The sample on pages 10–11 from my personal diary shows how you can use your diary.

KEY LONG-DISTANCE RUNS AND SPEED WORKOUTS

Use the chart on page 120 to record the important details of your long runs. You can analyze your improvement in distance, pace, and comfort as you get more fit. The data you gather here will be particularly valuable for your marathon training. Refer to the long-run guides on pages 156 and 165 to help you plan your long runs for races of 5k to the marathon.

The chart on page 121 can be used to record the key speed workouts that you complete. You can compare your times for the same or similar workouts to determine how sharp you are going into key races, or compare your times with previous training seasons. Refer to the Speed-Training Guide on page 160.

DAY
Mon
6/10
DATE

WEIGHT
169
54R
HEART RATE

COURSE/COMMENTS
I'm on my publicity tour for The Runner's Handbook

Houston
4 pm—Memorial Park Loop (dirt) from hotel 7½ at 8 pace
7:30 pm—Fun Run from bookstore—2 miles easy

Warm, humid

X WEIGHT TRAINING   X STRETCHING

TIME
60
8
PACE
MILES
9+
TO DATE

DAY
Tues
6/11
DATE

WEIGHT

130T
HEART RATE

COURSE/COMMENTS
San Francisco
4 pm—Marina to Golden Gate Bridge & Back—awesome view but banked and paved

Cool, windy

WEIGHT TRAINING   X STRETCHING

TIME
40
8
PACE
MILES
5
14
TO DATE

DAY
Wed
6/12
DATE

WEIGHT

HEART RATE

COURSE/COMMENTS
Portland
3 pm—from hotel along Willamette River—8+—nice views but banked pavement
7:30 pm—5+ from bookstore Fun Run—easy

65° low humidity

X WEIGHT TRAINING   X STRETCHING

TIME
8–8 1/2
PACE
MILES
14
28
TO DATE

DAY
Th
6/13
DATE

WEIGHT

HEART RATE

COURSE/COMMENTS
Seattle
3 pm—10 along Puget Sound from hotel—slow, tired

7:30 pm—2 very slow, bookstore Fun Run in Tacoma with view of Mt Rainier

Cool

WEIGHT TRAINING   X STRETCHING

TIME
85
8 1/2
PACE
MILES
12
40
TO DATE

DAY	COURSE/COMMENTS	TIME
Fri	Home!	27
6/14	But tired from flying, flying, flying	9
DATE		PACE
	6 pm—"Meadow 3" loop w/ Shelly-lynn—slow	
WEIGHT	30 min bike indoor re=4 miles	MILES
		3
130T 60R		43
HEART RATE	☐ WEIGHT TRAINING X STRETCHING	TO DATE

DAY	COURSE/COMMENTS	TIME
Sat	Back to work	
6/15	11 am—Central Park Reservoir 2 loops from bookstore Fun	8
DATE	Run—4+	PACE
	4 pm—"Rock 5" with Shelly-lynn—easy	
WEIGHT		MILES
		9
		52
HEART RATE	X WEIGHT TRAINING X STRETCHING	TO DATE

DAY	COURSE/COMMENTS	TIME
Sun	9 am—Pocantico Hills Crest 10 mile w/ Westchester Track	1:24
6/16	Club group, Paul & Shelly-lynn. Held back.	8:20
DATE	1:24:15 + ½ mile before & after	PACE
	(1:16 last time)	
WEIGHT		MILES
168	Still tired	11
	Very hot & hilly from book tour	63
HEART RATE	☐ WEIGHT TRAINING X STRETCHING	TO DATE

WEEKLY SUMMARY

Longest Run	11	Survived RHB book tour with third straight 60+ week!
Total # Workouts		
Runs	11-7 days	No speed tng for week. All runs 8 pace & slower
Speed training	0	
Cross training	1	But a success
Weight training	3	
Stretching	7	

WEEKLY TOTAL

63

1020/
42.5 avg.
YEAR TO DATE

WEEK OF:

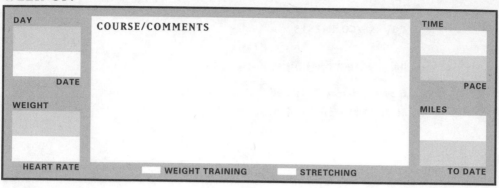

DAY

DATE

WEIGHT

HEART RATE

COURSE/COMMENTS

☐ WEIGHT TRAINING   ☐ STRETCHING

TIME

PACE

MILES

TO DATE

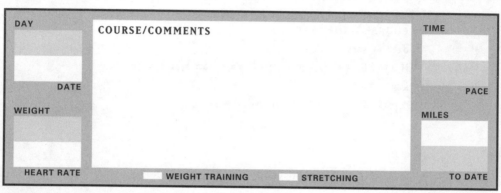

DAY

DATE

WEIGHT

HEART RATE

COURSE/COMMENTS

☐ WEIGHT TRAINING   ☐ STRETCHING

TIME

PACE

MILES

TO DATE

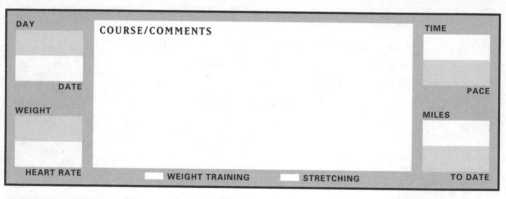

DAY

DATE

WEIGHT

HEART RATE

COURSE/COMMENTS

☐ WEIGHT TRAINING   ☐ STRETCHING

TIME

PACE

MILES

TO DATE

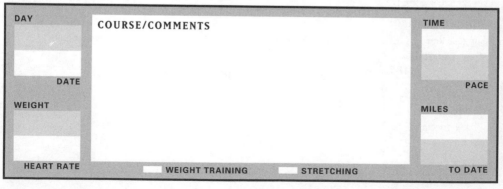

DAY

DATE

WEIGHT

HEART RATE

COURSE/COMMENTS

☐ WEIGHT TRAINING   ☐ STRETCHING

TIME

PACE

MILES

TO DATE

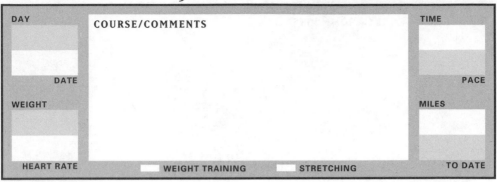

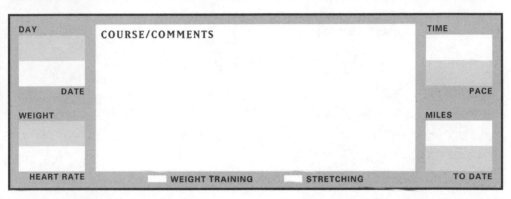

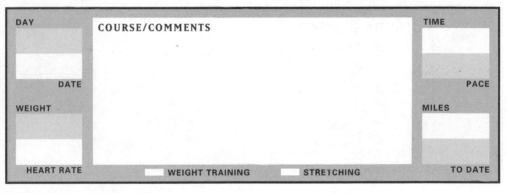

WEEKLY SUMMARY

Longest Run _____

Total # Workouts

Runs _____

Speed training _____

Cross training _____

Weight training_____

Stretching _____

WEEKLY TOTAL

YEAR TO DATE

WEEK OF:

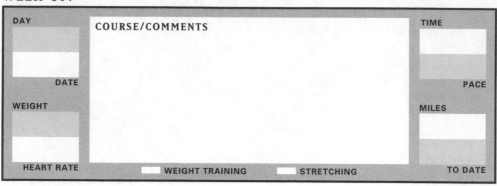

DAY

DATE

WEIGHT

HEART RATE

COURSE/COMMENTS

WEIGHT TRAINING   STRETCHING

TIME

PACE

MILES

TO DATE

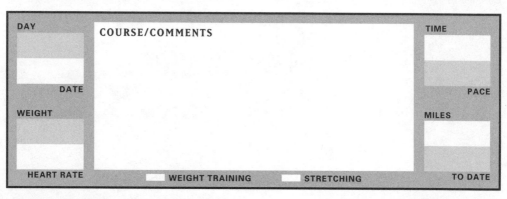

DAY

DATE

WEIGHT

HEART RATE

COURSE/COMMENTS

WEIGHT TRAINING   STRETCHING

TIME

PACE

MILES

TO DATE

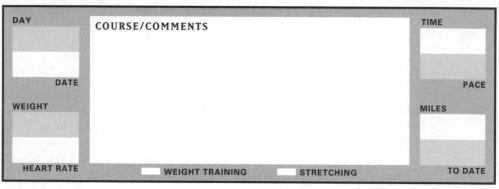

DAY

DATE

WEIGHT

HEART RATE

COURSE/COMMENTS

WEIGHT TRAINING   STRETCHING

TIME

PACE

MILES

TO DATE

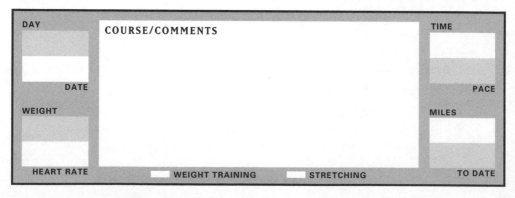

DAY

DATE

WEIGHT

HEART RATE

COURSE/COMMENTS

WEIGHT TRAINING   STRETCHING

TIME

PACE

MILES

TO DATE

DAY

DATE

WEIGHT

HEART RATE

COURSE/COMMENTS

□ WEIGHT TRAINING   □ STRETCHING

TIME

PACE

MILES

TO DATE

DAY

DATE

WEIGHT

HEART RATE

COURSE/COMMENTS

□ WEIGHT TRAINING   □ STRETCHING

TIME

PACE

MILES

TO DATE

DAY

DATE

WEIGHT

HEART RATE

COURSE/COMMENTS

□ WEIGHT TRAINING   □ STRETCHING

TIME

PACE

MILES

TO DATE

WEEKLY SUMMARY

Longest Run _____

Total # Workouts

Runs _____

Speed training _____

Cross training _____

Weight training_____

Stretching _____

WEEKLY TOTAL

YEAR TO DATE

WEEK OF:

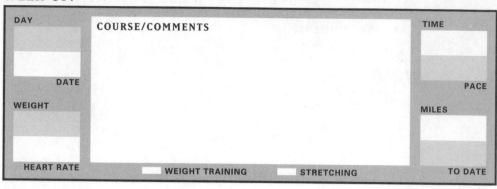

DAY

DATE

WEIGHT

HEART RATE

COURSE/COMMENTS

☐ WEIGHT TRAINING   ☐ STRETCHING

TIME

PACE

MILES

TO DATE

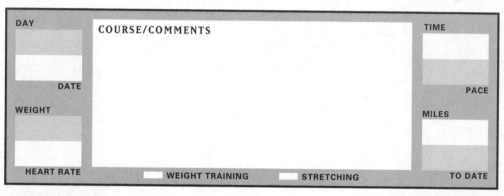

DAY

DATE

WEIGHT

HEART RATE

COURSE/COMMENTS

☐ WEIGHT TRAINING   ☐ STRETCHING

TIME

PACE

MILES

TO DATE

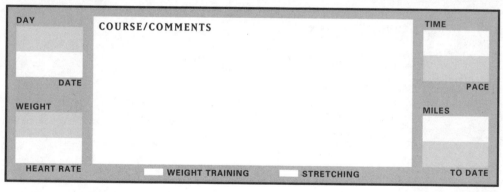

DAY

DATE

WEIGHT

HEART RATE

COURSE/COMMENTS

☐ WEIGHT TRAINING   ☐ STRETCHING

TIME

PACE

MILES

TO DATE

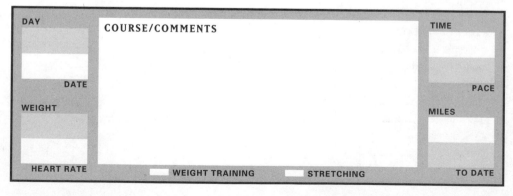

DAY

DATE

WEIGHT

HEART RATE

COURSE/COMMENTS

☐ WEIGHT TRAINING   ☐ STRETCHING

TIME

PACE

MILES

TO DATE

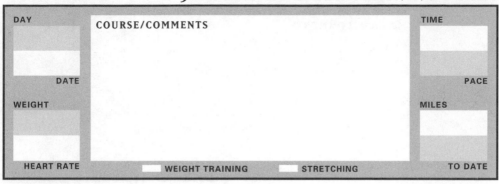

DAY	COURSE/COMMENTS		TIME
DATE			PACE
WEIGHT			MILES
HEART RATE	WEIGHT TRAINING	STRETCHING	TO DATE

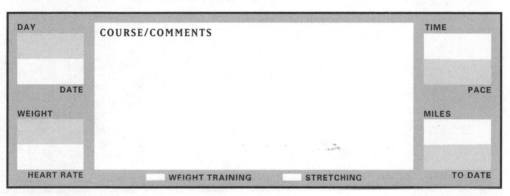

DAY	COURSE/COMMENTS		TIME
DATE			PACE
WEIGHT			MILES
HEART RATE	WEIGHT TRAINING	STRETCHING	TO DATE

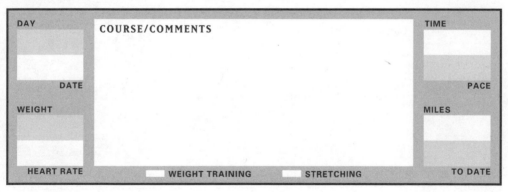

DAY	COURSE/COMMENTS		TIME
DATE			PACE
WEIGHT			MILES
HEART RATE	WEIGHT TRAINING	STRETCHING	TO DATE

WEEKLY SUMMARY

Longest Run _____

Total # Workouts

Runs _____

Speed training _____

Cross training _____

Weight training _____

Stretching _____

WEEKLY TOTAL

YEAR TO DATE

WEEK OF:

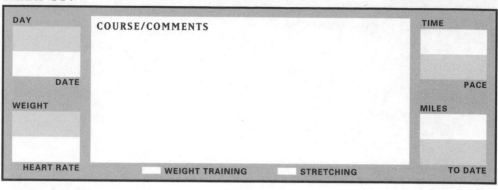

DAY

DATE

WEIGHT

HEART RATE

COURSE/COMMENTS

TIME

PACE

MILES

TO DATE

WEIGHT TRAINING STRETCHING

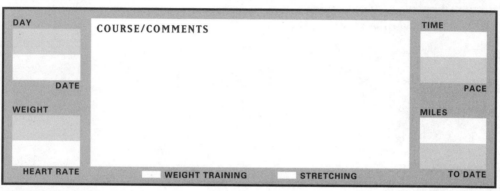

DAY

DATE

WEIGHT

HEART RATE

COURSE/COMMENTS

TIME

PACE

MILES

TO DATE

WEIGHT TRAINING STRETCHING

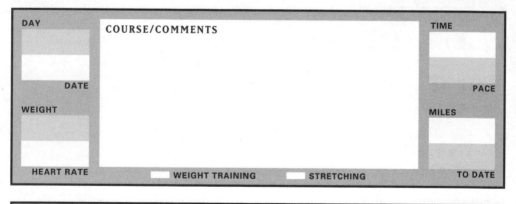

DAY

DATE

WEIGHT

HEART RATE

COURSE/COMMENTS

TIME

PACE

MILES

TO DATE

WEIGHT TRAINING STRETCHING

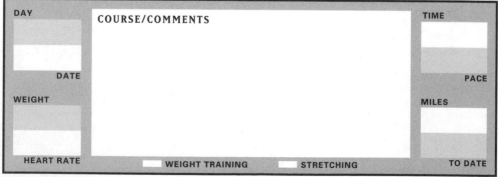

DAY

DATE

WEIGHT

HEART RATE

COURSE/COMMENTS

TIME

PACE

MILES

TO DATE

WEIGHT TRAINING STRETCHING

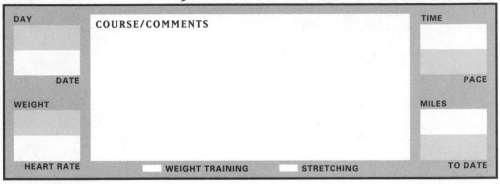

DAY

DATE

WEIGHT

HEART RATE

COURSE/COMMENTS

WEIGHT TRAINING   STRETCHING

TIME

PACE

MILES

TO DATE

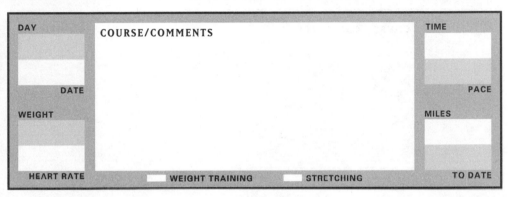

DAY

DATE

WEIGHT

HEART RATE

COURSE/COMMENTS

WEIGHT TRAINING   STRETCHING

TIME

PACE

MILES

TO DATE

DAY

DATE

WEIGHT

HEART RATE

COURSE/COMMENTS

WEIGHT TRAINING   STRETCHING

TIME

PACE

MILES

TO DATE

WEEKLY SUMMARY

Longest Run _____

Total # Workouts

Runs _____

Speed training _____

Cross training _____

Weight training _____

Stretching _____

WEEKLY TOTAL

YEAR TO DATE

WEEK OF:

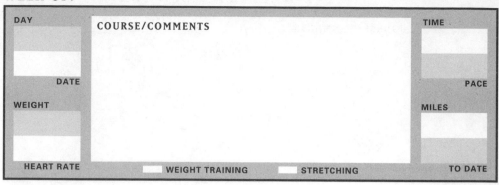

DAY

DATE

WEIGHT

HEART RATE

COURSE/COMMENTS

WEIGHT TRAINING   STRETCHING

TIME

PACE

MILES

TO DATE

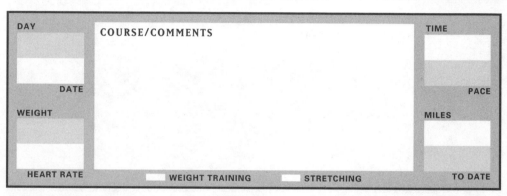

DAY

DATE

WEIGHT

HEART RATE

COURSE/COMMENTS

WEIGHT TRAINING   STRETCHING

TIME

PACE

MILES

TO DATE

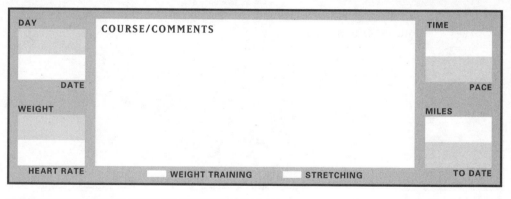

DAY

DATE

WEIGHT

HEART RATE

COURSE/COMMENTS

WEIGHT TRAINING   STRETCHING

TIME

PACE

MILES

TO DATE

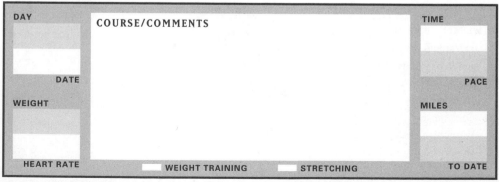

DAY

DATE

WEIGHT

HEART RATE

COURSE/COMMENTS

WEIGHT TRAINING   STRETCHING

TIME

PACE

MILES

TO DATE

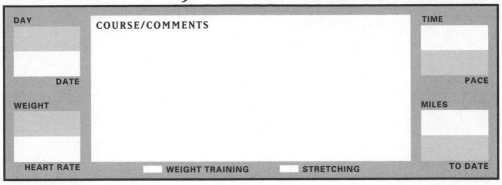

DAY

DATE

WEIGHT

HEART RATE

COURSE/COMMENTS

WEIGHT TRAINING   STRETCHING

TIME

PACE

MILES

TO DATE

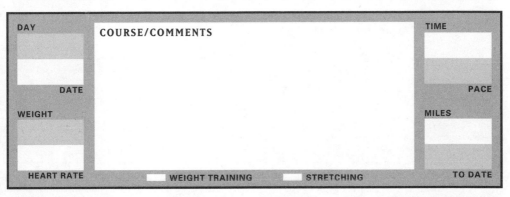

DAY

DATE

WEIGHT

HEART RATE

COURSE/COMMENTS

WEIGHT TRAINING   STRETCHING

TIME

PACE

MILES

TO DATE

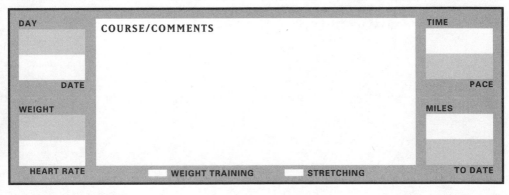

DAY

DATE

WEIGHT

HEART RATE

COURSE/COMMENTS

WEIGHT TRAINING   STRETCHING

TIME

PACE

MILES

TO DATE

WEEKLY SUMMARY

Longest Run _____

Total # Workouts

Runs _____

Speed training _____

Cross training _____

Weight training _____

Stretching _____

WEEKLY TOTAL

YEAR TO DATE

WEEK OF:

DAY

DATE

WEIGHT

HEART RATE

COURSE/COMMENTS

☐ WEIGHT TRAINING   ☐ STRETCHING

TIME

PACE

MILES

TO DATE

DAY

DATE

WEIGHT

HEART RATE

COURSE/COMMENTS

☐ WEIGHT TRAINING   ☐ STRETCHING

TIME

PACE

MILES

TO DATE

DAY

DATE

WEIGHT

HEART RATE

COURSE/COMMENTS

☐ WEIGHT TRAINING   ☐ STRETCHING

TIME

PACE

MILES

TO DATE

DAY

DATE

WEIGHT

HEART RATE

COURSE/COMMENTS

☐ WEIGHT TRAINING   ☐ STRETCHING

TIME

PACE

MILES

TO DATE

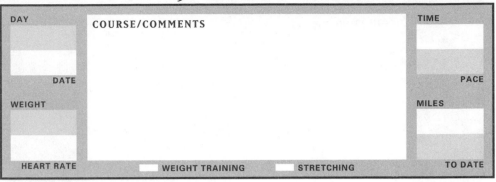

DAY

DATE

WEIGHT

HEART RATE

COURSE/COMMENTS

WEIGHT TRAINING   STRETCHING

TIME

PACE

MILES

TO DATE

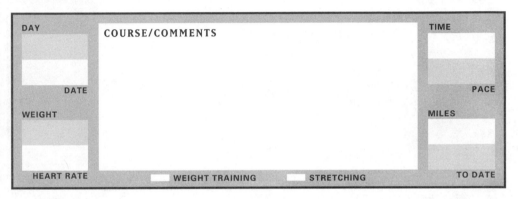

DAY

DATE

WEIGHT

HEART RATE

COURSE/COMMENTS

WEIGHT TRAINING   STRETCHING

TIME

PACE

MILES

TO DATE

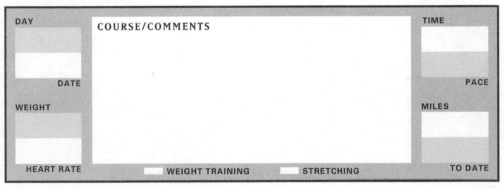

DAY

DATE

WEIGHT

HEART RATE

COURSE/COMMENTS

WEIGHT TRAINING   STRETCHING

TIME

PACE

MILES

TO DATE

WEEKLY SUMMARY

Longest Run _____

Total # Workouts

Runs _____

Speed training _____

Cross training _____

Weight training _____

Stretching _____

WEEKLY TOTAL

YEAR TO DATE

WEEK OF:

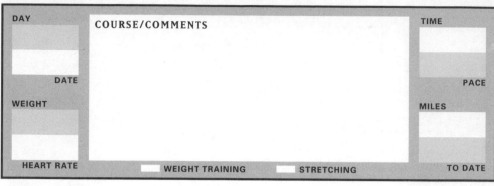

DAY

DATE

WEIGHT

HEART RATE

COURSE/COMMENTS

WEIGHT TRAINING   STRETCHING

TIME

PACE

MILES

TO DATE

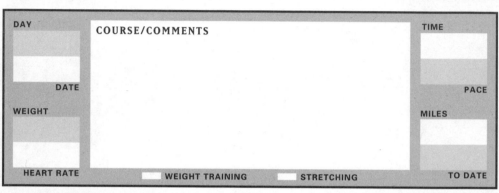

DAY

DATE

WEIGHT

HEART RATE

COURSE/COMMENTS

WEIGHT TRAINING   STRETCHING

TIME

PACE

MILES

TO DATE

DAY

DATE

WEIGHT

HEART RATE

COURSE/COMMENTS

WEIGHT TRAINING   STRETCHING

TIME

PACE

MILES

TO DATE

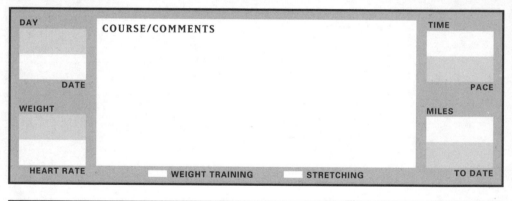

DAY

DATE

WEIGHT

HEART RATE

COURSE/COMMENTS

WEIGHT TRAINING   STRETCHING

TIME

PACE

MILES

TO DATE

24

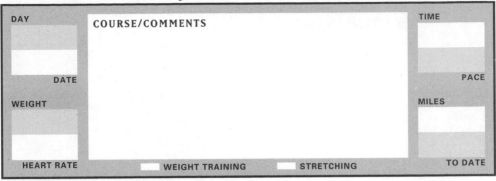

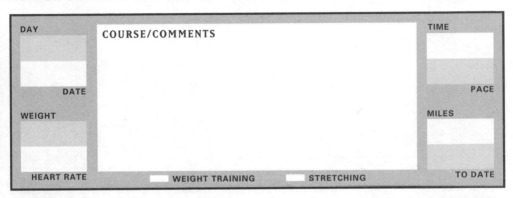

DAY

COURSE/COMMENTS

TIME

DATE

PACE

WEIGHT

MILES

HEART RATE   WEIGHT TRAINING   STRETCHING   TO DATE

WEEKLY SUMMARY

Longest Run _____

Total # Workouts

Runs   _____

Speed training _____

Cross training _____

Weight training_____

Stretching   _____

WEEKLY TOTAL

YEAR TO DATE

WEEK OF:

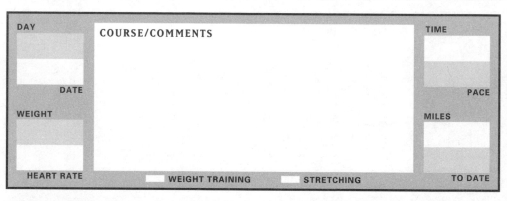

DAY

DATE

WEIGHT

HEART RATE

COURSE/COMMENTS

⬜ WEIGHT TRAINING   ⬜ STRETCHING

TIME

PACE

MILES

TO DATE

DAY

DATE

WEIGHT

HEART RATE

COURSE/COMMENTS

⬜ WEIGHT TRAINING   ⬜ STRETCHING

TIME

PACE

MILES

TO DATE

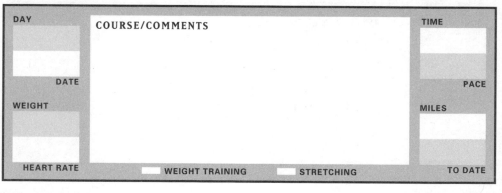

DAY

DATE

WEIGHT

HEART RATE

COURSE/COMMENTS

⬜ WEIGHT TRAINING   ⬜ STRETCHING

TIME

PACE

MILES

TO DATE

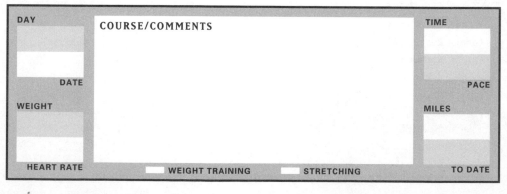

DAY

DATE

WEIGHT

HEART RATE

COURSE/COMMENTS

⬜ WEIGHT TRAINING   ⬜ STRETCHING

TIME

PACE

MILES

TO DATE

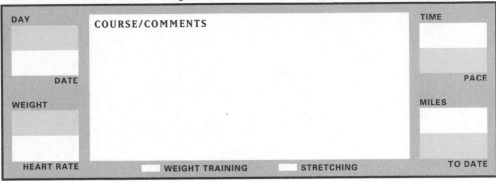

DAY	COURSE/COMMENTS		TIME
DATE			PACE
WEIGHT			MILES
HEART RATE	WEIGHT TRAINING	STRETCHING	TO DATE

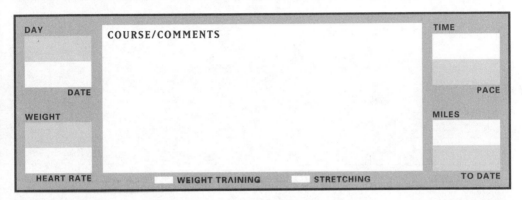

DAY	COURSE/COMMENTS		TIME
DATE			PACE
WEIGHT			MILES
HEART RATE	WEIGHT TRAINING	STRETCHING	TO DATE

DAY	COURSE/COMMENTS		TIME
DATE			PACE
WEIGHT			MILES
HEART RATE	WEIGHT TRAINING	STRETCHING	TO DATE

WEEKLY SUMMARY

Longest Run _____

Total # Workouts

Runs _____

Speed training _____

Cross training _____

Weight training _____

Stretching _____

WEEKLY TOTAL

YEAR TO DATE

WEEK OF:

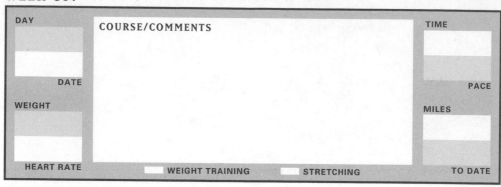

DAY

DATE

WEIGHT

HEART RATE

COURSE/COMMENTS

☐ WEIGHT TRAINING   ☐ STRETCHING

TIME

PACE

MILES

TO DATE

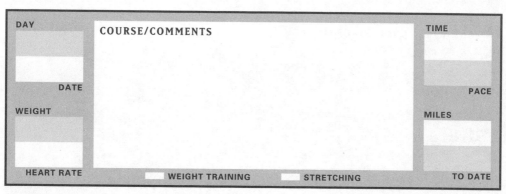

DAY

DATE

WEIGHT

HEART RATE

COURSE/COMMENTS

☐ WEIGHT TRAINING   ☐ STRETCHING

TIME

PACE

MILES

TO DATE

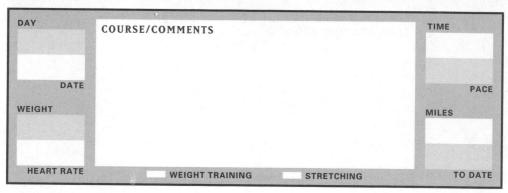

DAY

DATE

WEIGHT

HEART RATE

COURSE/COMMENTS

☐ WEIGHT TRAINING   ☐ STRETCHING

TIME

PACE

MILES

TO DATE

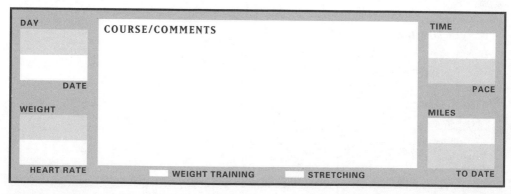

DAY

DATE

WEIGHT

HEART RATE

COURSE/COMMENTS

☐ WEIGHT TRAINING   ☐ STRETCHING

TIME

PACE

MILES

TO DATE

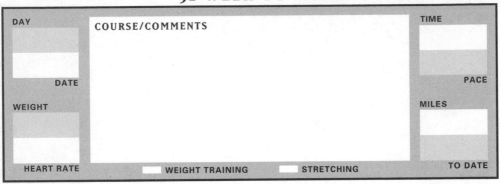

DAY

DATE

WEIGHT

HEART RATE

COURSE/COMMENTS

WEIGHT TRAINING   STRETCHING

TIME

PACE

MILES

TO DATE

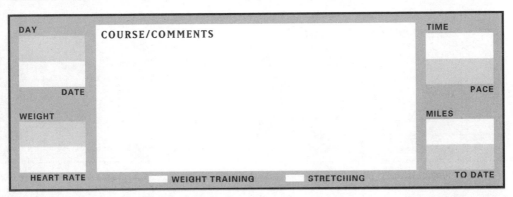

DAY

DATE

WEIGHT

HEART RATE

COURSE/COMMENTS

WEIGHT TRAINING   STRETCHING

TIME

PACE

MILES

TO DATE

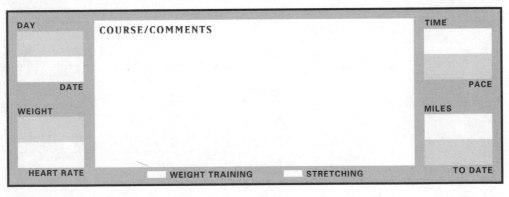

DAY

DATE

WEIGHT

HEART RATE

COURSE/COMMENTS

WEIGHT TRAINING   STRETCHING

TIME

PACE

MILES

TO DATE

WEEKLY SUMMARY

Longest Run _____

Total # Workouts

Runs _____

Speed training _____

Cross training _____

Weight training _____

Stretching _____

WEEKLY TOTAL

YEAR TO DATE

WEEK OF:

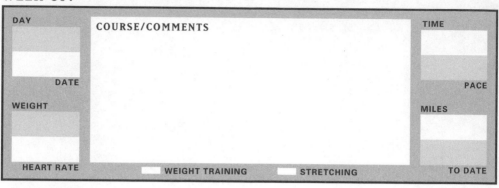

DAY

DATE

WEIGHT

HEART RATE

COURSE/COMMENTS

☐ WEIGHT TRAINING ☐ STRETCHING

TIME

PACE

MILES

TO DATE

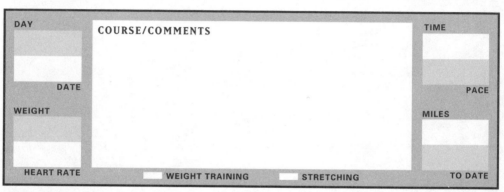

DAY

DATE

WEIGHT

HEART RATE

COURSE/COMMENTS

☐ WEIGHT TRAINING ☐ STRETCHING

TIME

PACE

MILES

TO DATE

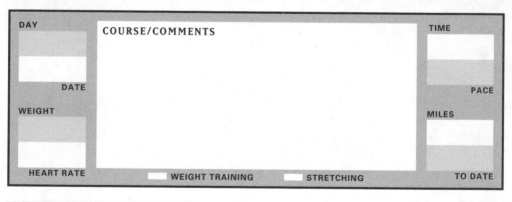

DAY

DATE

WEIGHT

HEART RATE

COURSE/COMMENTS

☐ WEIGHT TRAINING ☐ STRETCHING

TIME

PACE

MILES

TO DATE

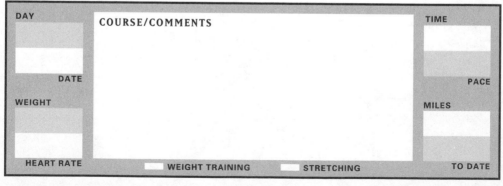

DAY

DATE

WEIGHT

HEART RATE

COURSE/COMMENTS

☐ WEIGHT TRAINING ☐ STRETCHING

TIME

PACE

MILES

TO DATE

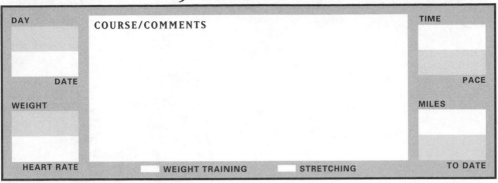

DAY

DATE

WEIGHT

HEART RATE

COURSE/COMMENTS

☐ WEIGHT TRAINING   ☐ STRETCHING

TIME

PACE

MILES

TO DATE

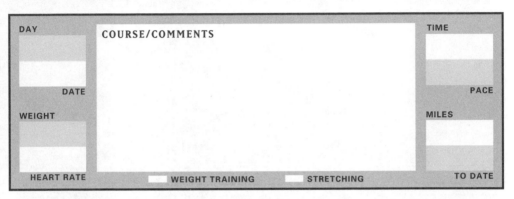

DAY

DATE

WEIGHT

HEART RATE

COURSE/COMMENTS

☐ WEIGHT TRAINING   ☐ STRETCHING

TIME

PACE

MILES

TO DATE

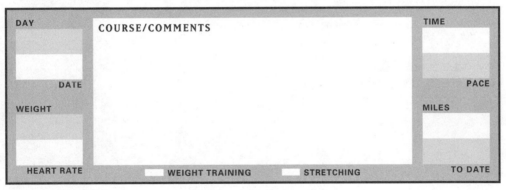

DAY

DATE

WEIGHT

HEART RATE

COURSE/COMMENTS

☐ WEIGHT TRAINING   ☐ STRETCHING

TIME

PACE

MILES

TO DATE

WEEKLY SUMMARY

Longest Run _____

Total # Workouts

Runs _____

Speed training _____

Cross training _____

Weight training _____

Stretching _____

WEEKLY TOTAL

YEAR TO DATE

WEEK OF:

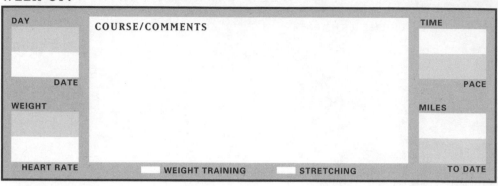

DAY
DATE
WEIGHT
HEART RATE

COURSE/COMMENTS

☐ WEIGHT TRAINING   ☐ STRETCHING

TIME
PACE
MILES
TO DATE

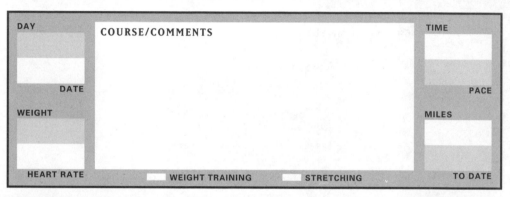

DAY
DATE
WEIGHT
HEART RATE

COURSE/COMMENTS

☐ WEIGHT TRAINING   ☐ STRETCHING

TIME
PACE
MILES
TO DATE

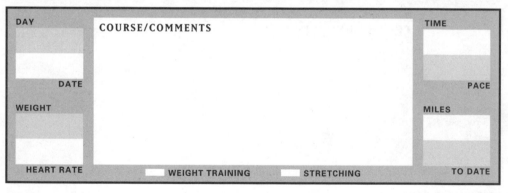

DAY
DATE
WEIGHT
HEART RATE

COURSE/COMMENTS

☐ WEIGHT TRAINING   ☐ STRETCHING

TIME
PACE
MILES
TO DATE

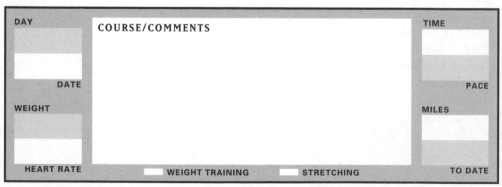

DAY
DATE
WEIGHT
HEART RATE

COURSE/COMMENTS

☐ WEIGHT TRAINING   ☐ STRETCHING

TIME
PACE
MILES
TO DATE

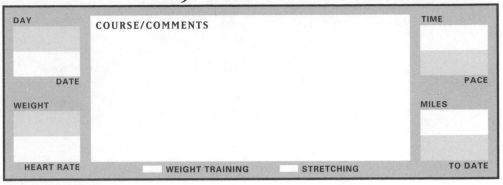

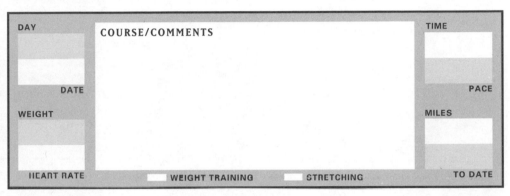

DAY	COURSE/COMMENTS	TIME
DATE		PACE
WEIGHT		MILES
HEART RATE	WEIGHT TRAINING STRETCHING	TO DATE

WEEKLY SUMMARY

Longest Run _____

Total # Workouts

Runs _____

Speed training _____

Cross training _____

Weight training _____

Stretching _____

WEEKLY TOTAL

YEAR TO DATE

WEEK OF:

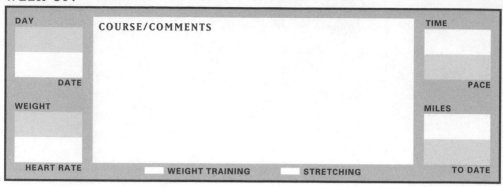

DAY

DATE

WEIGHT

HEART RATE

COURSE/COMMENTS

WEIGHT TRAINING   STRETCHING

TIME

PACE

MILES

TO DATE

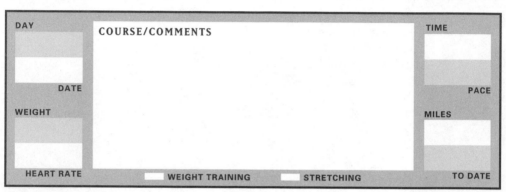

DAY

DATE

WEIGHT

HEART RATE

COURSE/COMMENTS

WEIGHT TRAINING   STRETCHING

TIME

PACE

MILES

TO DATE

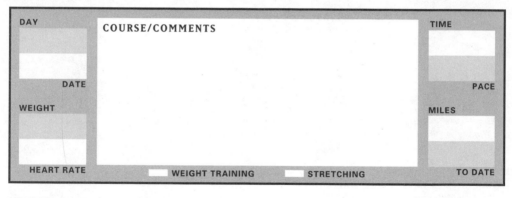

DAY

DATE

WEIGHT

HEART RATE

COURSE/COMMENTS

WEIGHT TRAINING   STRETCHING

TIME

PACE

MILES

TO DATE

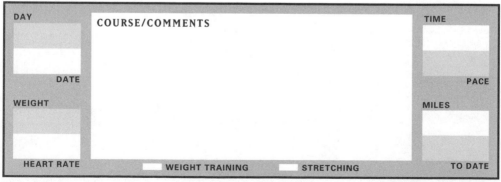

DAY

DATE

WEIGHT

HEART RATE

COURSE/COMMENTS

WEIGHT TRAINING   STRETCHING

TIME

PACE

MILES

TO DATE

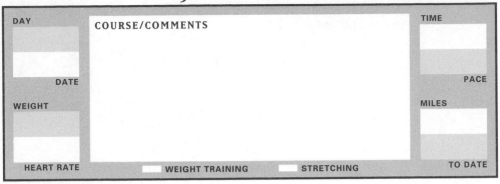

DAY

DATE

WEIGHT

HEART RATE

COURSE/COMMENTS

WEIGHT TRAINING   STRETCHING

TIME

PACE

MILES

TO DATE

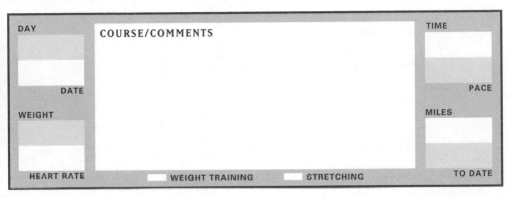

DAY

DATE

WEIGHT

HEART RATE

COURSE/COMMENTS

WEIGHT TRAINING   STRETCHING

TIME

PACE

MILES

TO DATE

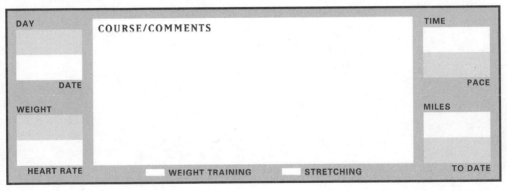

DAY

DATE

WEIGHT

HEART RATE

COURSE/COMMENTS

WEIGHT TRAINING   STRETCHING

TIME

PACE

MILES

TO DATE

WEEKLY SUMMARY

Longest Run _____

Total # Workouts

Runs _____

Speed training _____

Cross training _____

Weight training _____

Stretching _____

WEEKLY TOTAL

YEAR TO DATE

WEEK OF:

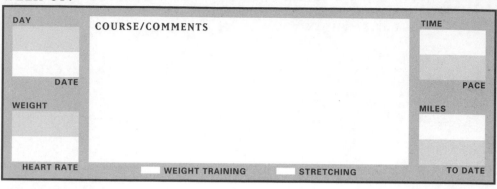

DAY

DATE

WEIGHT

HEART RATE

COURSE/COMMENTS

WEIGHT TRAINING   STRETCHING

TIME

PACE

MILES

TO DATE

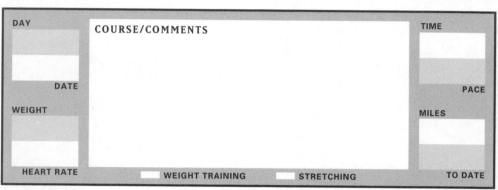

DAY

DATE

WEIGHT

HEART RATE

COURSE/COMMENTS

WEIGHT TRAINING   STRETCHING

TIME

PACE

MILES

TO DATE

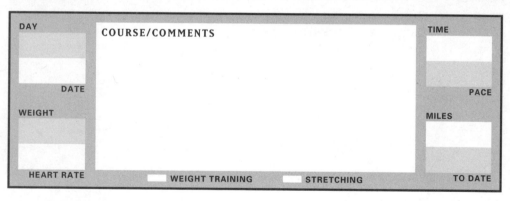

DAY

DATE

WEIGHT

HEART RATE

COURSE/COMMENTS

WEIGHT TRAINING   STRETCHING

TIME

PACE

MILES

TO DATE

DAY

DATE

WEIGHT

HEART RATE

COURSE/COMMENTS

WEIGHT TRAINING   STRETCHING

TIME

PACE

MILES

TO DATE

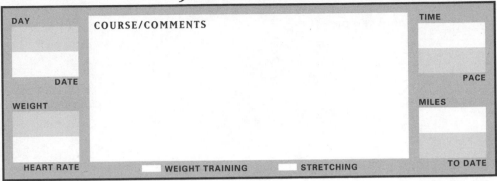

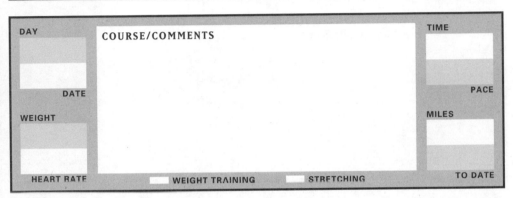

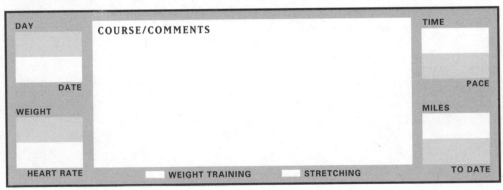

WEEKLY SUMMARY

Longest Run _____

Total # Workouts

Runs _____

Speed training _____

Cross training _____

Weight training _____

Stretching _____

WEEKLY TOTAL

YEAR TO DATE

WEEK OF:

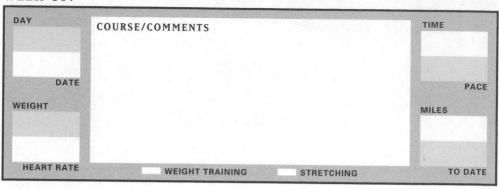

DAY

DATE

WEIGHT

HEART RATE

COURSE/COMMENTS

☐ WEIGHT TRAINING   ☐ STRETCHING

TIME

PACE

MILES

TO DATE

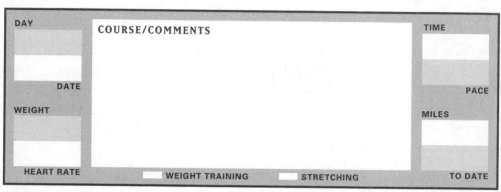

DAY

DATE

WEIGHT

HEART RATE

COURSE/COMMENTS

☐ WEIGHT TRAINING   ☐ STRETCHING

TIME

PACE

MILES

TO DATE

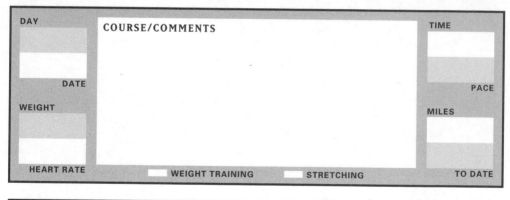

DAY

DATE

WEIGHT

HEART RATE

COURSE/COMMENTS

☐ WEIGHT TRAINING   ☐ STRETCHING

TIME

PACE

MILES

TO DATE

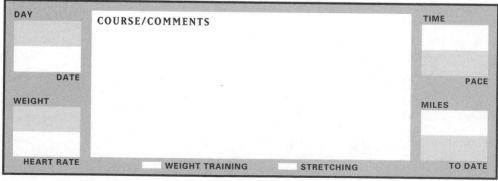

DAY

DATE

WEIGHT

HEART RATE

COURSE/COMMENTS

☐ WEIGHT TRAINING   ☐ STRETCHING

TIME

PACE

MILES

TO DATE

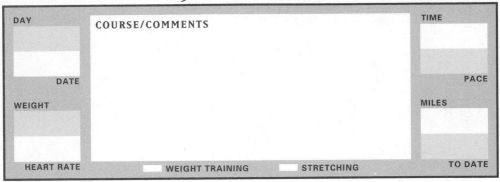

DAY

DATE

WEIGHT

HEART RATE

COURSE/COMMENTS

WEIGHT TRAINING   STRETCHING

TIME

PACE

MILES

TO DATE

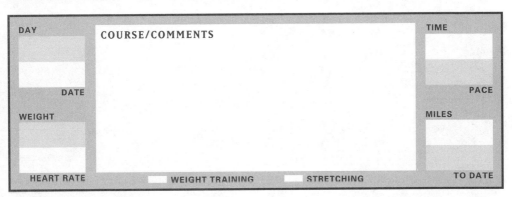

DAY

DATE

WEIGHT

HEART RATE

COURSE/COMMENTS

WEIGHT TRAINING   STRETCHING

TIME

PACE

MILES

TO DATE

DAY

DATE

WEIGHT

HEART RATE

COURSE/COMMENTS

WEIGHT TRAINING   STRETCHING

TIME

PACE

MILES

TO DATE

WEEKLY SUMMARY
Longest Run _____
Total # Workouts
  Runs   _____
  Speed training _____
  Cross training _____
  Weight training_____
  Stretching   _____

WEEKLY TOTAL

YEAR TO DATE

WEEK OF:

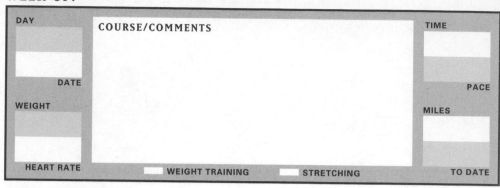

DAY

DATE

WEIGHT

HEART RATE

COURSE/COMMENTS

☐ WEIGHT TRAINING ☐ STRETCHING

TIME

PACE

MILES

TO DATE

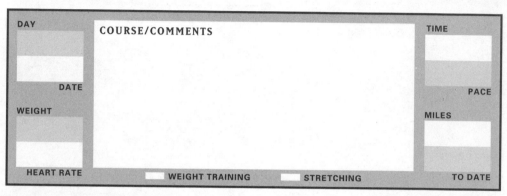

DAY

DATE

WEIGHT

HEART RATE

COURSE/COMMENTS

☐ WEIGHT TRAINING ☐ STRETCHING

TIME

PACE

MILES

TO DATE

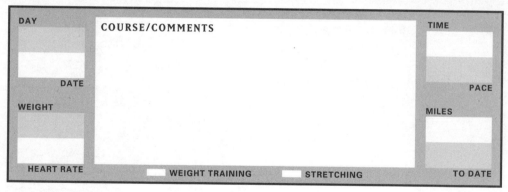

DAY

DATE

WEIGHT

HEART RATE

COURSE/COMMENTS

☐ WEIGHT TRAINING ☐ STRETCHING

TIME

PACE

MILES

TO DATE

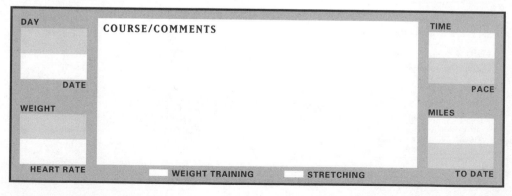

DAY

DATE

WEIGHT

HEART RATE

COURSE/COMMENTS

☐ WEIGHT TRAINING ☐ STRETCHING

TIME

PACE

MILES

TO DATE

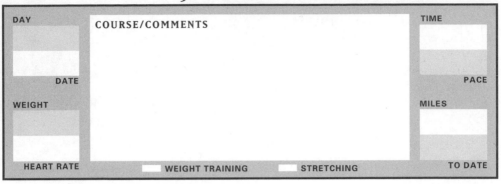

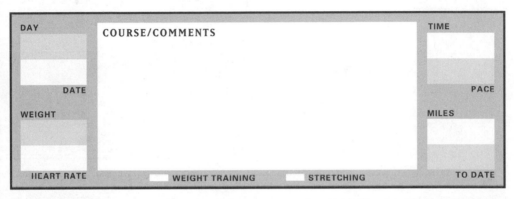

DAY	COURSE/COMMENTS	TIME
DATE		PACE
WEIGHT		MILES
HEART RATE	WEIGHT TRAINING STRETCHING	TO DATE

WEEKLY SUMMARY

Longest Run _____

Total # Workouts

Runs _____

Speed training _____

Cross training _____

Weight training_____

Stretching _____

WEEKLY TOTAL

YEAR TO DATE

WEEK OF:

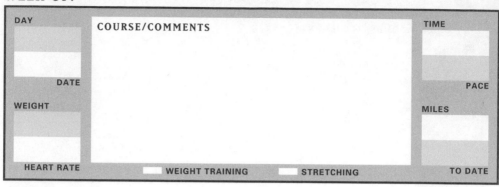

DAY

DATE

WEIGHT

HEART RATE

COURSE/COMMENTS

WEIGHT TRAINING   STRETCHING

TIME

PACE

MILES

TO DATE

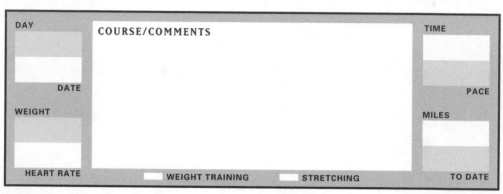

DAY

DATE

WEIGHT

HEART RATE

COURSE/COMMENTS

WEIGHT TRAINING   STRETCHING

TIME

PACE

MILES

TO DATE

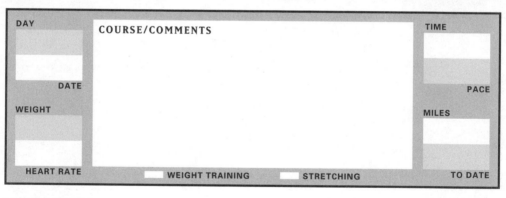

DAY

DATE

WEIGHT

HEART RATE

COURSE/COMMENTS

WEIGHT TRAINING   STRETCHING

TIME

PACE

MILES

TO DATE

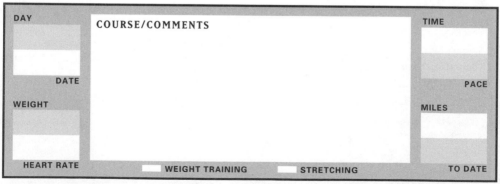

DAY

DATE

WEIGHT

HEART RATE

COURSE/COMMENTS

WEIGHT TRAINING   STRETCHING

TIME

PACE

MILES

TO DATE

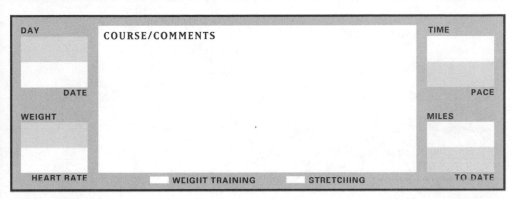

DAY	COURSE/COMMENTS	TIME
DATE		PACE
WEIGHT		MILES
HEART RATE	WEIGHT TRAINING STRETCHING	TO DATE

DAY	COURSE/COMMENTS	TIME
DATE		PACE
WEIGHT		MILES
HEART RATE	WEIGHT TRAINING STRETCHING	TO DATE

DAY	COURSE/COMMENTS	TIME
DATE		PACE
WEIGHT		MILES
HEART RATE	WEIGHT TRAINING STRETCHING	TO DATE

WEEKLY SUMMARY

Longest Run _____

Total # Workouts

Runs _____

Speed training _____

Cross training _____

Weight training _____

Stretching _____

WEEKLY TOTAL

YEAR TO DATE

WEEK OF:

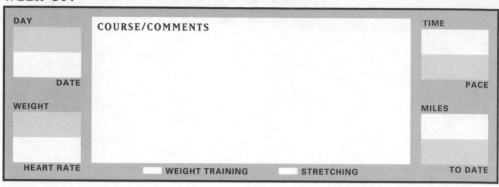

DAY

DATE

WEIGHT

HEART RATE

COURSE/COMMENTS

TIME

PACE

MILES

WEIGHT TRAINING   STRETCHING

TO DATE

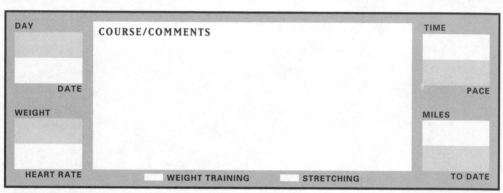

DAY

DATE

WEIGHT

HEART RATE

COURSE/COMMENTS

TIME

PACE

MILES

WEIGHT TRAINING   STRETCHING

TO DATE

DAY

DATE

WEIGHT

HEART RATE

COURSE/COMMENTS

TIME

PACE

MILES

WEIGHT TRAINING   STRETCHING

TO DATE

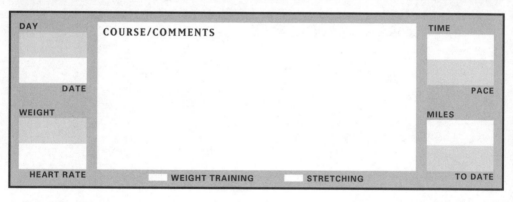

DAY

DATE

WEIGHT

HEART RATE

COURSE/COMMENTS

TIME

PACE

MILES

WEIGHT TRAINING   STRETCHING

TO DATE

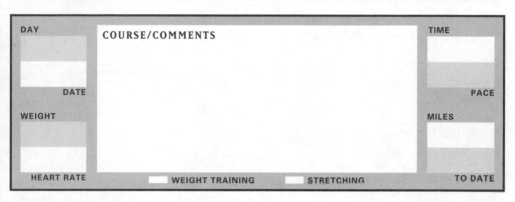

DAY

DATE

WEIGHT

HEART RATE

COURSE/COMMENTS

WEIGHT TRAINING   STRETCHING

TIME

PACE

MILES

TO DATE

DAY

DATE

WEIGHT

HEART RATE

COURSE/COMMENTS

WEIGHT TRAINING   STRETCHING

TIME

PACE

MILES

TO DATE

DAY

DATE

WEIGHT

HEART RATE

COURSE/COMMENTS

WEIGHT TRAINING   STRETCHING

TIME

PACE

MILES

TO DATE

WEEKLY SUMMARY

Longest Run _____

Total # Workouts

Runs _____

Speed training _____

Cross training _____

Weight training _____

Stretching _____

WEEKLY TOTAL

YEAR TO DATE

WEEK OF:

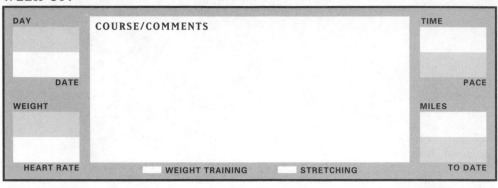

DAY

DATE

WEIGHT

HEART RATE

COURSE/COMMENTS

☐ WEIGHT TRAINING ☐ STRETCHING

TIME

PACE

MILES

TO DATE

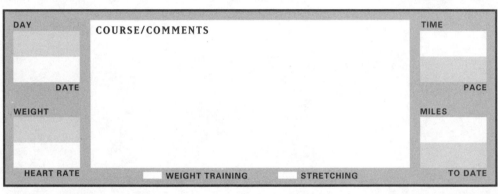

DAY

DATE

WEIGHT

HEART RATE

COURSE/COMMENTS

☐ WEIGHT TRAINING ☐ STRETCHING

TIME

PACE

MILES

TO DATE

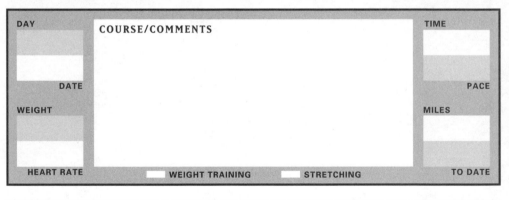

DAY

DATE

WEIGHT

HEART RATE

COURSE/COMMENTS

☐ WEIGHT TRAINING ☐ STRETCHING

TIME

PACE

MILES

TO DATE

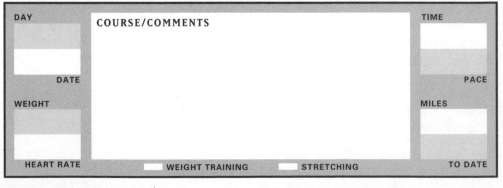

DAY

DATE

WEIGHT

HEART RATE

COURSE/COMMENTS

☐ WEIGHT TRAINING ☐ STRETCHING

TIME

PACE

MILES

TO DATE

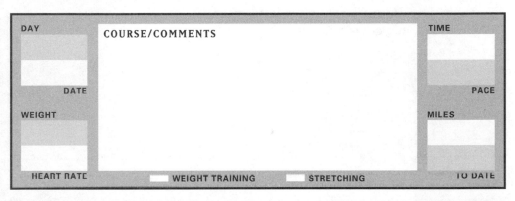

DAY	COURSE/COMMENTS	TIME
DATE		PACE
WEIGHT		MILES
HEART RATE	WEIGHT TRAINING STRETCHING	TO DATE

DAY	COURSE/COMMENTS	TIME
DATE		PACE
WEIGHT		MILES
HEART RATE	WEIGHT TRAINING STRETCHING	TO DATE

DAY	COURSE/COMMENTS	TIME
DATE		PACE
WEIGHT		MILES
HEART RATE	WEIGHT TRAINING STRETCHING	TO DATE

WEEKLY SUMMARY

Longest Run _____

Total # Workouts

Runs _____

Speed training _____

Cross training _____

Weight training _____

Stretching _____

WEEKLY TOTAL

YEAR TO DATE

WEEK OF:

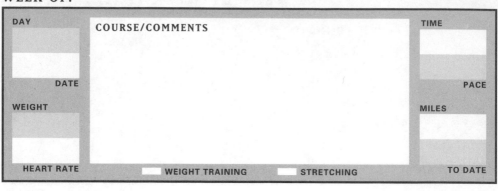

DAY

DATE

WEIGHT

HEART RATE

COURSE/COMMENTS

☐ WEIGHT TRAINING ☐ STRETCHING

TIME

PACE

MILES

TO DATE

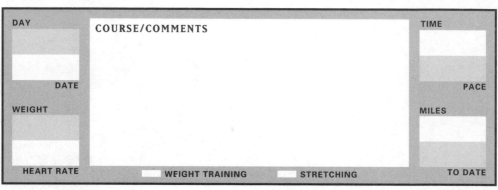

DAY

DATE

WEIGHT

HEART RATE

COURSE/COMMENTS

☐ WEIGHT TRAINING ☐ STRETCHING

TIME

PACE

MILES

TO DATE

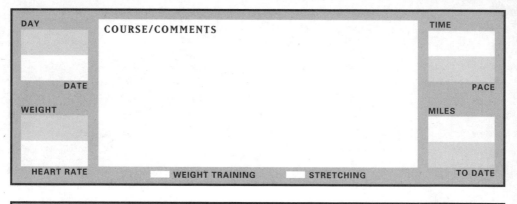

DAY

DATE

WEIGHT

HEART RATE

COURSE/COMMENTS

☐ WEIGHT TRAINING ☐ STRETCHING

TIME

PACE

MILES

TO DATE

DAY

DATE

WEIGHT

HEART RATE

COURSE/COMMENTS

☐ WEIGHT TRAINING ☐ STRETCHING

TIME

PACE

MILES

TO DATE

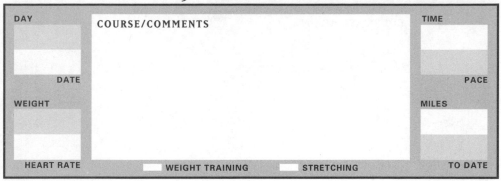

DAY

DATE

WEIGHT

HEART RATE

COURSE/COMMENTS

WEIGHT TRAINING STRETCHING

TIME

PACE

MILES

TO DATE

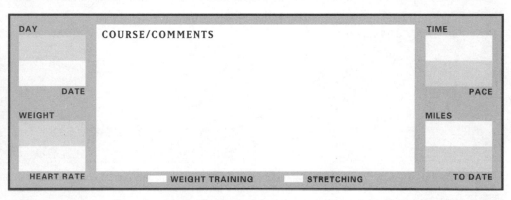

DAY

DATE

WEIGHT

HEART RATE

COURSE/COMMENTS

WEIGHT TRAINING STRETCHING

TIME

PACE

MILES

TO DATE

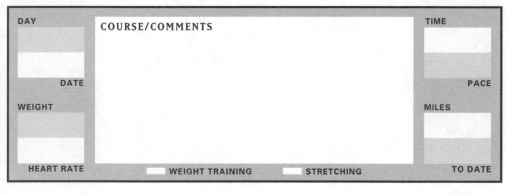

DAY

DATE

WEIGHT

HEART RATE

COURSE/COMMENTS

WEIGHT TRAINING STRETCHING

TIME

PACE

MILES

TO DATE

WEEKLY SUMMARY

Longest Run _____

Total # Workouts

Runs _____

Speed training _____

Cross training _____

Weight training _____

Stretching _____

WEEKLY TOTAL

YEAR TO DATE

WEEK OF:

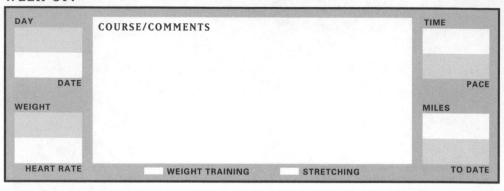

DAY

DATE

WEIGHT

HEART RATE

COURSE/COMMENTS

☐ WEIGHT TRAINING   ☐ STRETCHING

TIME

PACE

MILES

TO DATE

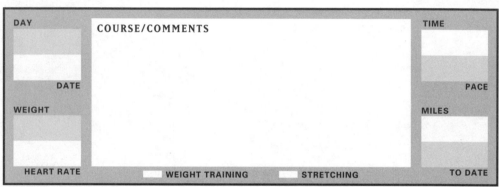

DAY

DATE

WEIGHT

HEART RATE

COURSE/COMMENTS

☐ WEIGHT TRAINING   ☐ STRETCHING

TIME

PACE

MILES

TO DATE

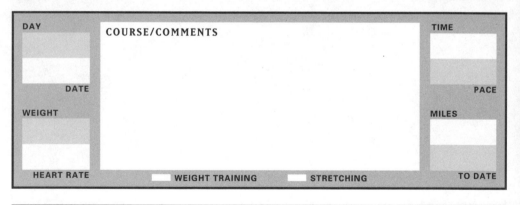

DAY

DATE

WEIGHT

HEART RATE

COURSE/COMMENTS

☐ WEIGHT TRAINING   ☐ STRETCHING

TIME

PACE

MILES

TO DATE

DAY

DATE

WEIGHT

HEART RATE

COURSE/COMMENTS

☐ WEIGHT TRAINING   ☐ STRETCHING

TIME

PACE

MILES

TO DATE

DAY	COURSE/COMMENTS	TIME
DATE		PACE
WEIGHT		MILES
HEART RATE	WEIGHT TRAINING STRETCHING	TO DATE

DAY	COURSE/COMMENTS	TIME
DATE		PACE
WEIGHT		MILES
HEART RATE	WEIGHT TRAINING STRETCHING	TO DATE

DAY	COURSE/COMMENTS	TIME
DATE		PACE
WEIGHT		MILES
HEART RATE	WEIGHT TRAINING STRETCHING	TO DATE

WEEKLY SUMMARY
Longest Run _____
Total # Workouts
  Runs _____
  Speed training _____
  Cross training _____
  Weight training_____
  Stretching _____

WEEKLY TOTAL

YEAR TO DATE

WEEK OF:

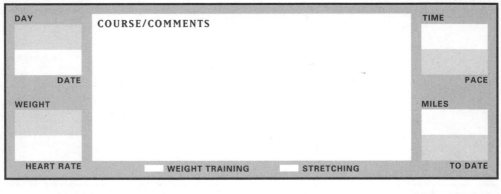

DAY

DATE

WEIGHT

HEART RATE

COURSE/COMMENTS

WEIGHT TRAINING   STRETCHING

TIME

PACE

MILES

TO DATE

DAY

DATE

WEIGHT

HEART RATE

COURSE/COMMENTS

WEIGHT TRAINING   STRETCHING

TIME

PACE

MILES

TO DATE

DAY

DATE

WEIGHT

HEART RATE

COURSE/COMMENTS

WEIGHT TRAINING   STRETCHING

TIME

PACE

MILES

TO DATE

DAY

DATE

WEIGHT

HEART RATE

COURSE/COMMENTS

WEIGHT TRAINING   STRETCHING

TIME

PACE

MILES

TO DATE

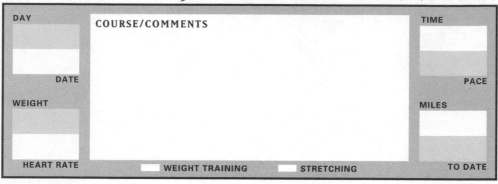

DAY

DATE

WEIGHT

HEART RATE

COURSE/COMMENTS

WEIGHT TRAINING   STRETCHING

TIME

PACE

MILES

TO DATE

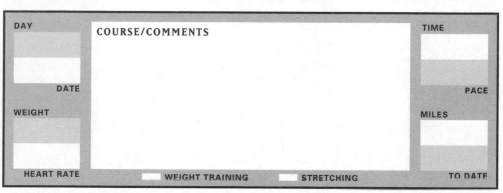

DAY

DATE

WEIGHT

HEART RATE

COURSE/COMMENTS

WEIGHT TRAINING   STRETCHING

TIME

PACE

MILES

TO DATE

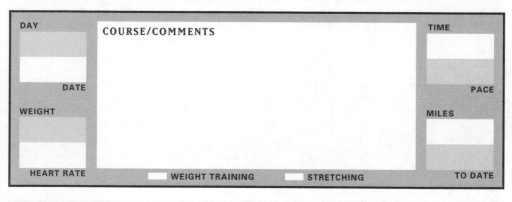

DAY

DATE

WEIGHT

HEART RATE

COURSE/COMMENTS

WEIGHT TRAINING   STRETCHING

TIME

PACE

MILES

TO DATE

WEEKLY SUMMARY

Longest Run _____

Total # Workouts

Runs _____

Speed training _____

Cross training _____

Weight training _____

Stretching _____

WEEKLY TOTAL

YEAR TO DATE

WEEK OF:

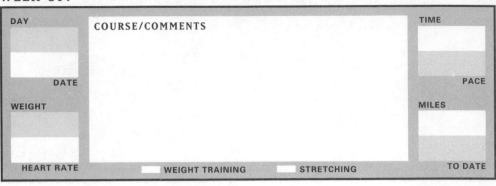

DAY
DATE
WEIGHT
HEART RATE

COURSE/COMMENTS

☐ WEIGHT TRAINING ☐ STRETCHING

TIME
PACE
MILES
TO DATE

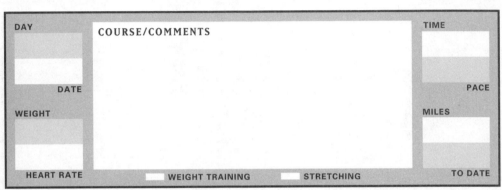

DAY
DATE
WEIGHT
HEART RATE

COURSE/COMMENTS

☐ WEIGHT TRAINING ☐ STRETCHING

TIME
PACE
MILES
TO DATE

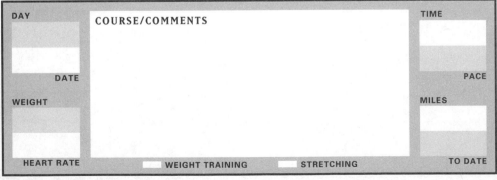

DAY
DATE
WEIGHT
HEART RATE

COURSE/COMMENTS

☐ WEIGHT TRAINING ☐ STRETCHING

TIME
PACE
MILES
TO DATE

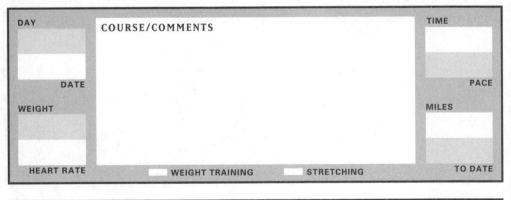

DAY
DATE
WEIGHT
HEART RATE

COURSE/COMMENTS

☐ WEIGHT TRAINING ☐ STRETCHING

TIME
PACE
MILES
TO DATE

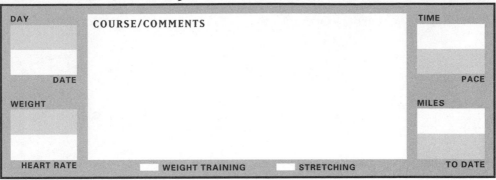

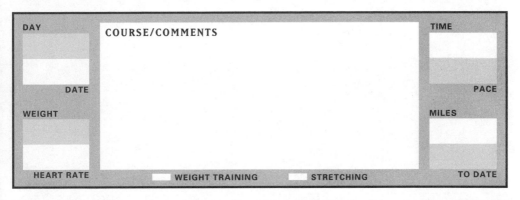

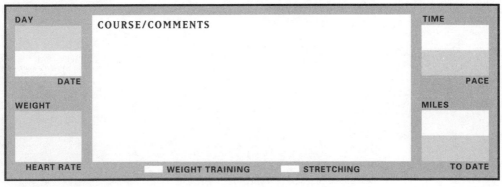

WEEKLY SUMMARY

Longest Run _____

Total # Workouts

Runs _____

Speed training _____

Cross training _____

Weight training _____

Stretching _____

WEEKLY TOTAL

YEAR TO DATE

WEEK OF:

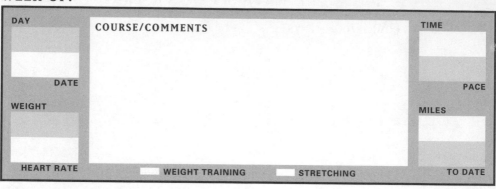

DAY

DATE

WEIGHT

HEART RATE

COURSE/COMMENTS

☐ WEIGHT TRAINING   ☐ STRETCHING

TIME

PACE

MILES

TO DATE

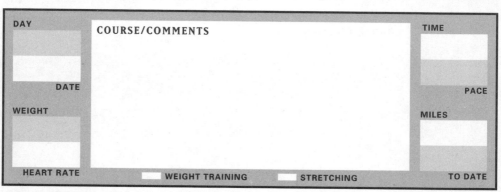

DAY

DATE

WEIGHT

HEART RATE

COURSE/COMMENTS

☐ WEIGHT TRAINING   ☐ STRETCHING

TIME

PACE

MILES

TO DATE

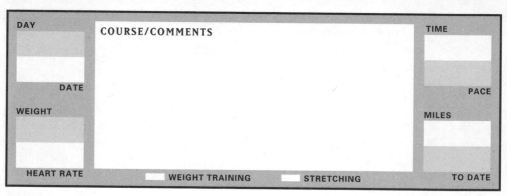

DAY

DATE

WEIGHT

HEART RATE

COURSE/COMMENTS

☐ WEIGHT TRAINING   ☐ STRETCHING

TIME

PACE

MILES

TO DATE

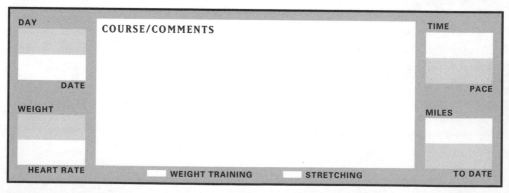

DAY

DATE

WEIGHT

HEART RATE

COURSE/COMMENTS

☐ WEIGHT TRAINING   ☐ STRETCHING

TIME

PACE

MILES

TO DATE

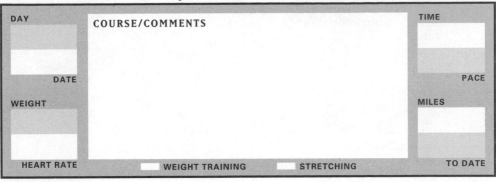

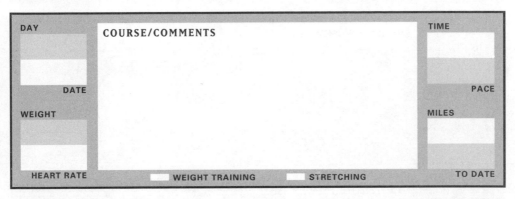

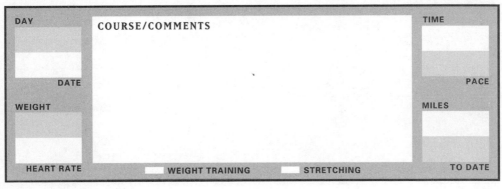

WEEKLY SUMMARY

Longest Run _____

Total # Workouts

Runs _____

Speed training _____

Cross training _____

Weight training _____

Stretching _____

WEEKLY TOTAL

YEAR TO DATE

WEEK OF:

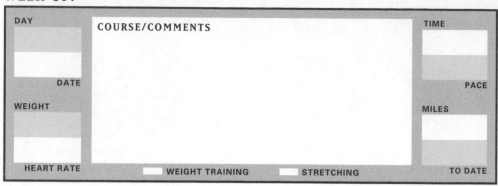

DAY

DATE

WEIGHT

HEART RATE

COURSE/COMMENTS

☐ WEIGHT TRAINING   ☐ STRETCHING

TIME

PACE

MILES

TO DATE

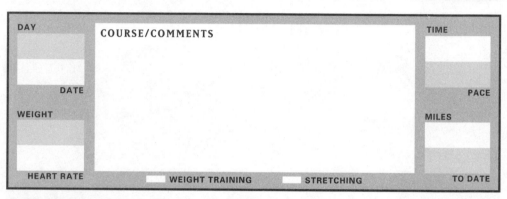

DAY

DATE

WEIGHT

HEART RATE

COURSE/COMMENTS

☐ WEIGHT TRAINING   ☐ STRETCHING

TIME

PACE

MILES

TO DATE

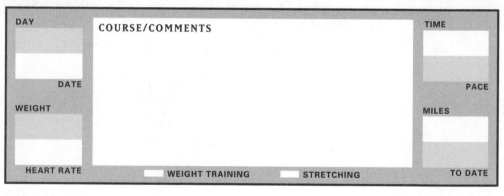

DAY

DATE

WEIGHT

HEART RATE

COURSE/COMMENTS

☐ WEIGHT TRAINING   ☐ STRETCHING

TIME

PACE

MILES

TO DATE

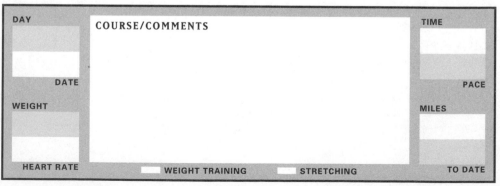

DAY

DATE

WEIGHT

HEART RATE

COURSE/COMMENTS

☐ WEIGHT TRAINING   ☐ STRETCHING

TIME

PACE

MILES

TO DATE

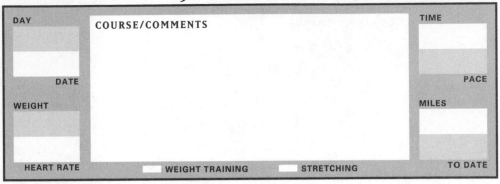

DAY	COURSE/COMMENTS	TIME
DATE		PACE
WEIGHT		MILES
HEART RATE	WEIGHT TRAINING ☐ STRETCHING ☐	TO DATE

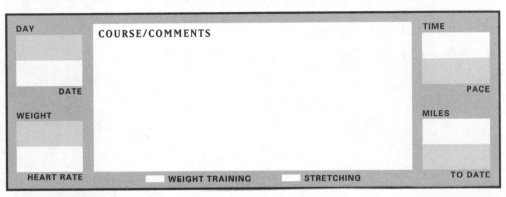

DAY	COURSE/COMMENTS	TIME
DATE		PACE
WEIGHT		MILES
HEART RATE	WEIGHT TRAINING ☐ STRETCHING ☐	TO DATE

DAY	COURSE/COMMENTS	TIME
DATE		PACE
WEIGHT		MILES
HEART RATE	WEIGHT TRAINING ☐ STRETCHING ☐	TO DATE

WEEKLY SUMMARY

Longest Run _____

Total # Workouts

Runs _____

Speed training _____

Cross training _____

Weight training _____

Stretching _____

WEEKLY TOTAL

YEAR TO DATE

WEEK OF:

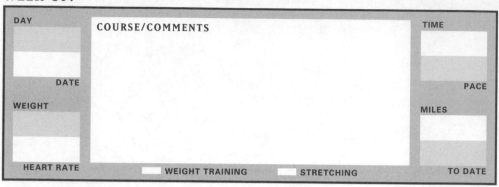

DAY

DATE

WEIGHT

HEART RATE

COURSE/COMMENTS

WEIGHT TRAINING   STRETCHING

TIME

PACE

MILES

TO DATE

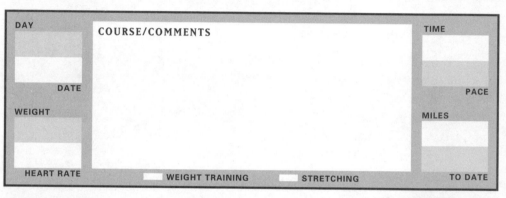

DAY

DATE

WEIGHT

HEART RATE

COURSE/COMMENTS

WEIGHT TRAINING   STRETCHING

TIME

PACE

MILES

TO DATE

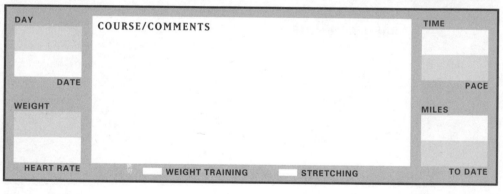

DAY

DATE

WEIGHT

HEART RATE

COURSE/COMMENTS

WEIGHT TRAINING   STRETCHING

TIME

PACE

MILES

TO DATE

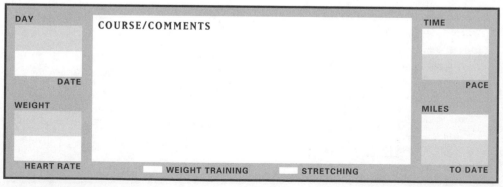

DAY

DATE

WEIGHT

HEART RATE

COURSE/COMMENTS

WEIGHT TRAINING   STRETCHING

TIME

PACE

MILES

TO DATE

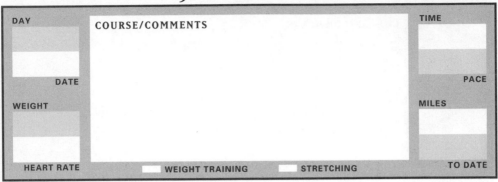

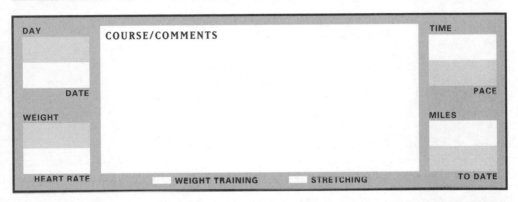

DAY	COURSE/COMMENTS	TIME
DATE		PACE
WEIGHT		MILES
HEART RATE	WEIGHT TRAINING STRETCHING	TO DATE

WEEKLY SUMMARY

Longest Run _____

Total # Workouts

Runs _____

Speed training _____

Cross training _____

Weight training _____

Stretching _____

WEEKLY TOTAL

YEAR TO DATE

WEEK OF:

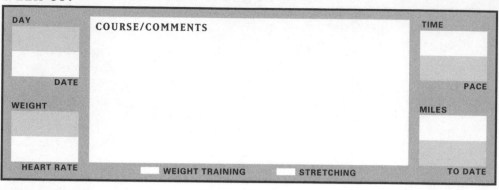

DAY

DATE

WEIGHT

HEART RATE

COURSE/COMMENTS

WEIGHT TRAINING   STRETCHING

TIME

PACE

MILES

TO DATE

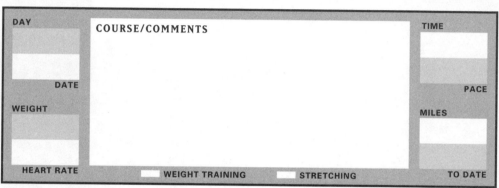

DAY

DATE

WEIGHT

HEART RATE

COURSE/COMMENTS

WEIGHT TRAINING   STRETCHING

TIME

PACE

MILES

TO DATE

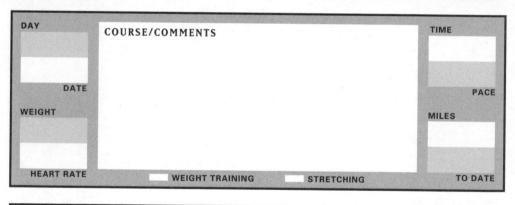

DAY

DATE

WEIGHT

HEART RATE

COURSE/COMMENTS

WEIGHT TRAINING   STRETCHING

TIME

PACE

MILES

TO DATE

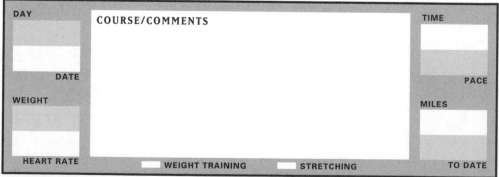

DAY

DATE

WEIGHT

HEART RATE

COURSE/COMMENTS

WEIGHT TRAINING   STRETCHING

TIME

PACE

MILES

TO DATE

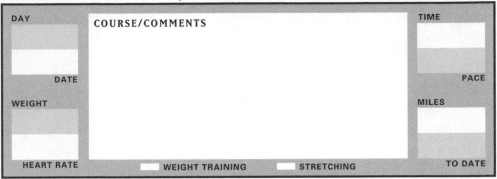

DAY	COURSE/COMMENTS		TIME
DATE			PACE
WEIGHT			MILES
HEART RATE	WEIGHT TRAINING	STRETCHING	TO DATE

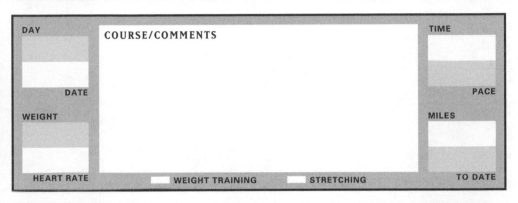

DAY	COURSE/COMMENTS		TIME
DATE			PACE
WEIGHT			MILES
HEART RATE	WEIGHT TRAINING	STRETCHING	TO DATE

DAY	COURSE/COMMENTS		TIME
DATE			PACE
WEIGHT			MILES
HEART RATE	WEIGHT TRAINING	STRETCHING	TO DATE

WEEKLY SUMMARY

Longest Run _____

Total # Workouts

Runs _____

Speed training _____

Cross training _____

Weight training _____

Stretching _____

WEEKLY TOTAL

YEAR TO DATE

WEEK OF:

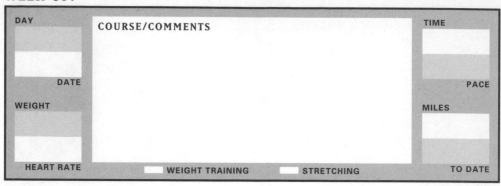

DAY

DATE

WEIGHT

HEART RATE

COURSE/COMMENTS

WEIGHT TRAINING ☐ STRETCHING ☐

TIME

PACE

MILES

TO DATE

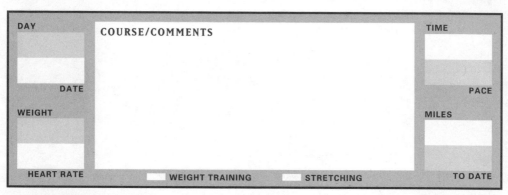

DAY

DATE

WEIGHT

HEART RATE

COURSE/COMMENTS

WEIGHT TRAINING ☐ STRETCHING ☐

TIME

PACE

MILES

TO DATE

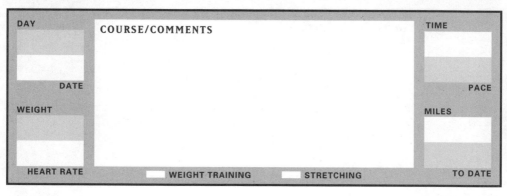

DAY

DATE

WEIGHT

HEART RATE

COURSE/COMMENTS

WEIGHT TRAINING ☐ STRETCHING ☐

TIME

PACE

MILES

TO DATE

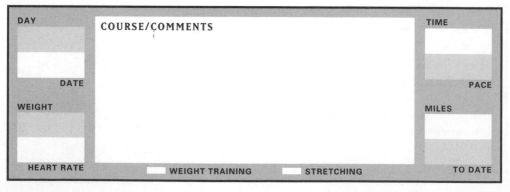

DAY

DATE

WEIGHT

HEART RATE

COURSE/COMMENTS

WEIGHT TRAINING ☐ STRETCHING ☐

TIME

PACE

MILES

TO DATE

64

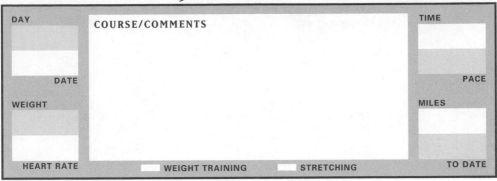

DAY

DATE

WEIGHT

HEART RATE

COURSE/COMMENTS

WEIGHT TRAINING   STRETCHING

TIME

PACE

MILES

TO DATE

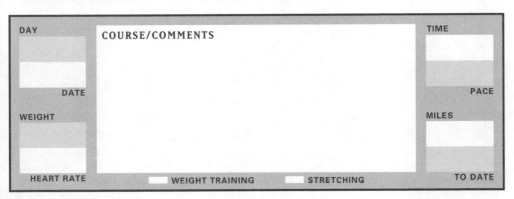

DAY

DATE

WEIGHT

HEART RATE

COURSE/COMMENTS

WEIGHT TRAINING   STRETCHING

TIME

PACE

MILES

TO DATE

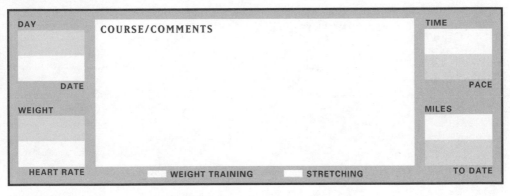

DAY

DATE

WEIGHT

HEART RATE

COURSE/COMMENTS

WEIGHT TRAINING   STRETCHING

TIME

PACE

MILES

TO DATE

WEEKLY SUMMARY

Longest Run _____

Total # Workouts

Runs _____

Speed training _____

Cross training _____

Weight training _____

Stretching _____

WEEKLY TOTAL

YEAR TO DATE

WEEK OF:

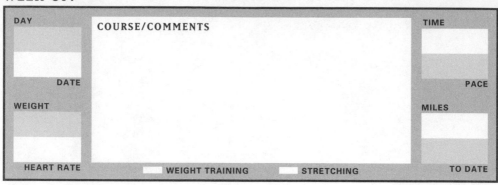

DAY

DATE

WEIGHT

HEART RATE

COURSE/COMMENTS

WEIGHT TRAINING   STRETCHING

TIME

PACE

MILES

TO DATE

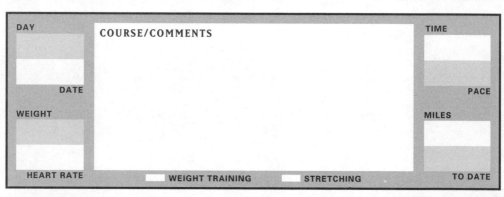

DAY

DATE

WEIGHT

HEART RATE

COURSE/COMMENTS

WEIGHT TRAINING   STRETCHING

TIME

PACE

MILES

TO DATE

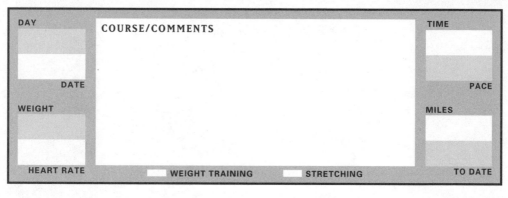

DAY

DATE

WEIGHT

HEART RATE

COURSE/COMMENTS

WEIGHT TRAINING   STRETCHING

TIME

PACE

MILES

TO DATE

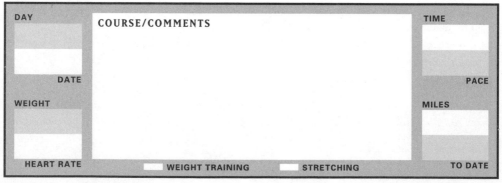

DAY

DATE

WEIGHT

HEART RATE

COURSE/COMMENTS

WEIGHT TRAINING   STRETCHING

TIME

PACE

MILES

TO DATE

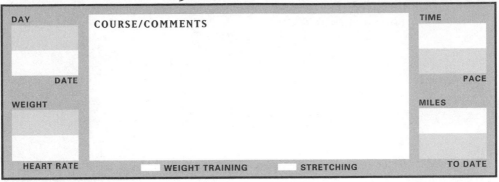

DAY

DATE

WEIGHT

HEART RATE

COURSE/COMMENTS

WEIGHT TRAINING   STRETCHING

TIME

PACE

MILES

TO DATE

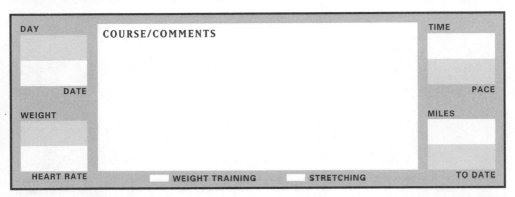

DAY

DATE

WEIGHT

HEART RATE

COURSE/COMMENTS

WEIGHT TRAINING   STRETCHING

TIME

PACE

MILES

TO DATE

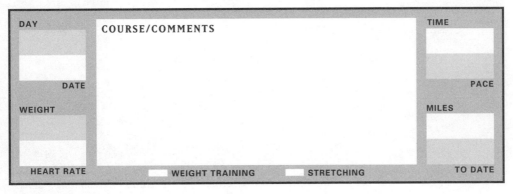

DAY

DATE

WEIGHT

HEART RATE

COURSE/COMMENTS

WEIGHT TRAINING   STRETCHING

TIME

PACE

MILES

TO DATE

WEEKLY SUMMARY

Longest Run _____

Total # Workouts

Runs _____

Speed training _____

Cross training _____

Weight training_____

Stretching _____

WEEKLY TOTAL

YEAR TO DATE

WEEK OF:

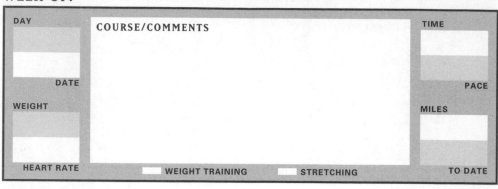

DAY
DATE
WEIGHT
HEART RATE

COURSE/COMMENTS

WEIGHT TRAINING   STRETCHING

TIME
PACE
MILES
TO DATE

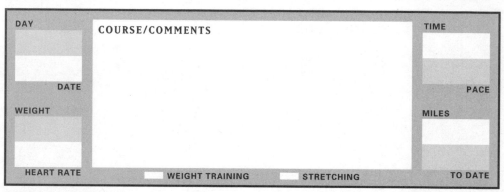

DAY
DATE
WEIGHT
HEART RATE

COURSE/COMMENTS

WEIGHT TRAINING   STRETCHING

TIME
PACE
MILES
TO DATE

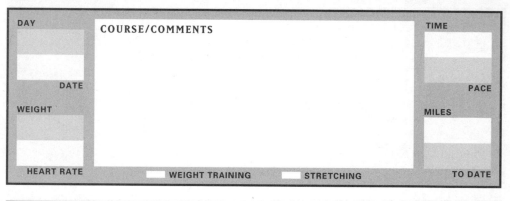

DAY
DATE
WEIGHT
HEART RATE

COURSE/COMMENTS

WEIGHT TRAINING   STRETCHING

TIME
PACE
MILES
TO DATE

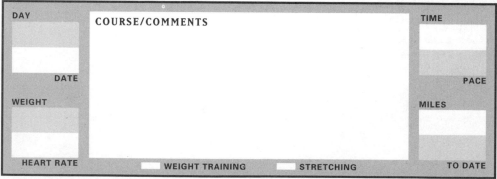

DAY
DATE
WEIGHT
HEART RATE

COURSE/COMMENTS

WEIGHT TRAINING   STRETCHING

TIME
PACE
MILES
TO DATE

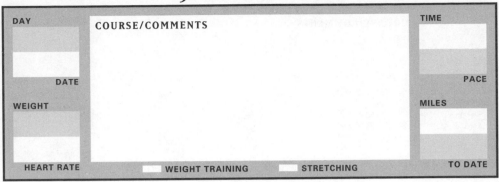

DAY

DATE

WEIGHT

HEART RATE

COURSE/COMMENTS

TIME

PACE

MILES

TO DATE

WEIGHT TRAINING   STRETCHING

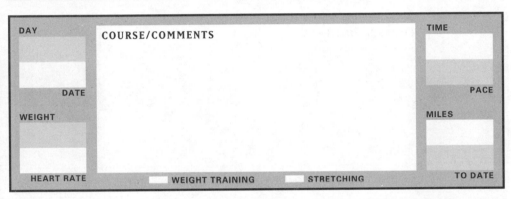

DAY

DATE

WEIGHT

HEART RATE

COURSE/COMMENTS

TIME

PACE

MILES

TO DATE

WEIGHT TRAINING   STRETCHING

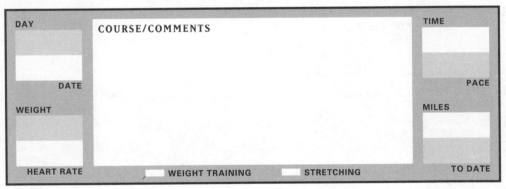

DAY

DATE

WEIGHT

HEART RATE

COURSE/COMMENTS

TIME

PACE

MILES

TO DATE

WEIGHT TRAINING   STRETCHING

WEEKLY SUMMARY

Longest Run _____

Total # Workouts

Runs _____

Speed training _____

Cross training _____

Weight training _____

Stretching _____

WEEKLY TOTAL

YEAR TO DATE

WEEK OF:

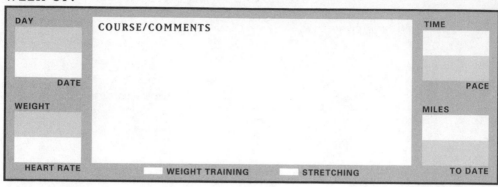

DAY

DATE

WEIGHT

HEART RATE

COURSE/COMMENTS

WEIGHT TRAINING

STRETCHING

TIME

PACE

MILES

TO DATE

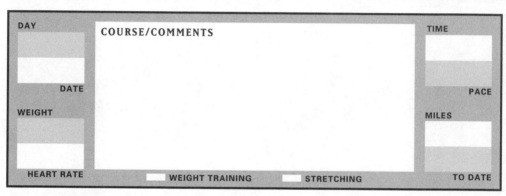

DAY

DATE

WEIGHT

HEART RATE

COURSE/COMMENTS

WEIGHT TRAINING

STRETCHING

TIME

PACE

MILES

TO DATE

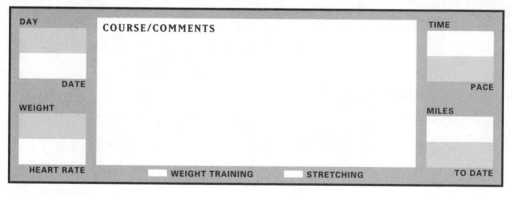

DAY

DATE

WEIGHT

HEART RATE

COURSE/COMMENTS

WEIGHT TRAINING

STRETCHING

TIME

PACE

MILES

TO DATE

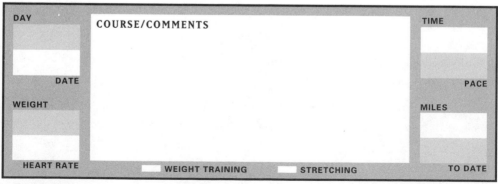

DAY

DATE

WEIGHT

HEART RATE

COURSE/COMMENTS

WEIGHT TRAINING

STRETCHING

TIME

PACE

MILES

TO DATE

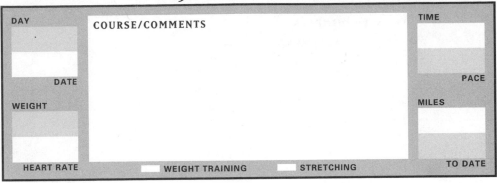

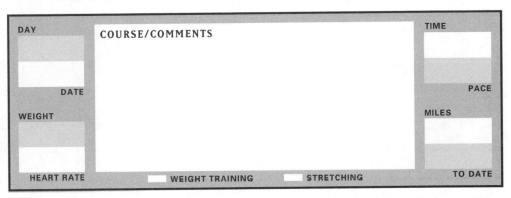

DAY	COURSE/COMMENTS	TIME
DATE		PACE
WEIGHT		MILES
HEART RATE	WEIGHT TRAINING STRETCHING	TO DATE

DAY	COURSE/COMMENTS	TIME
DATE		PACE
WEIGHT		MILES
HEART RATE	WEIGHT TRAINING STRETCHING	TO DATE

WEEKLY SUMMARY

Longest Run _____

Total # Workouts

Runs _____

Speed training _____

Cross training _____

Weight training _____

Stretching _____

WEEKLY TOTAL

YEAR TO DATE

WEEK OF:

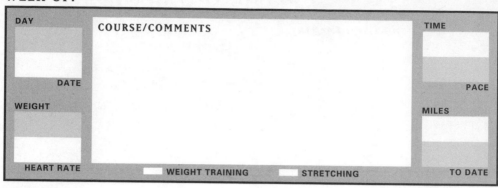

DAY

DATE

WEIGHT

HEART RATE

COURSE/COMMENTS

WEIGHT TRAINING   STRETCHING

TIME

PACE

MILES

TO DATE

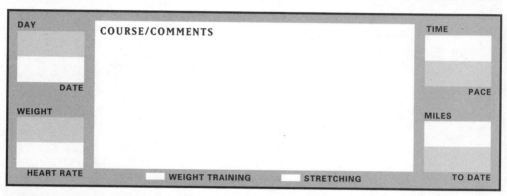

DAY

DATE

WEIGHT

HEART RATE

COURSE/COMMENTS

WEIGHT TRAINING   STRETCHING

TIME

PACE

MILES

TO DATE

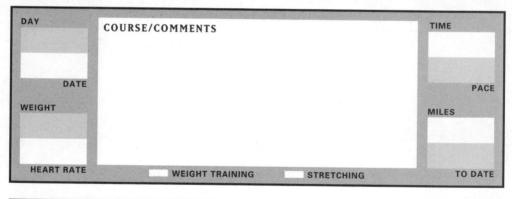

DAY

DATE

WEIGHT

HEART RATE

COURSE/COMMENTS

WEIGHT TRAINING   STRETCHING

TIME

PACE

MILES

TO DATE

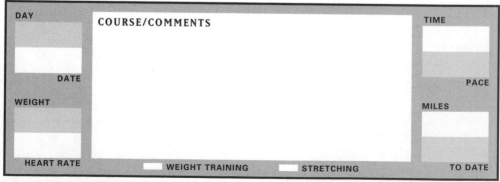

DAY

DATE

WEIGHT

HEART RATE

COURSE/COMMENTS

WEIGHT TRAINING   STRETCHING

TIME

PACE

MILES

TO DATE

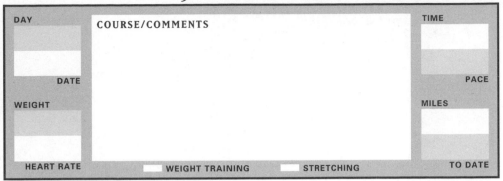

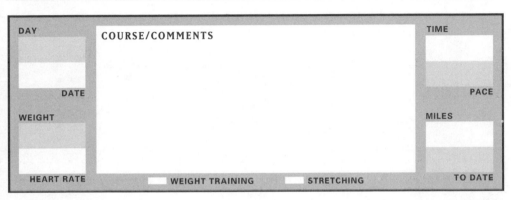

DAY	COURSE/COMMENTS	TIME
DATE		PACE
WEIGHT		MILES
HEART RATE	WEIGHT TRAINING STRETCHING	TO DATE

WEEKLY SUMMARY

Longest Run _____

Total # Workouts

   Runs _____

   Speed training _____

   Cross training _____

   Weight training _____

   Stretching _____

WEEKLY TOTAL

YEAR TO DATE

WEEK OF:

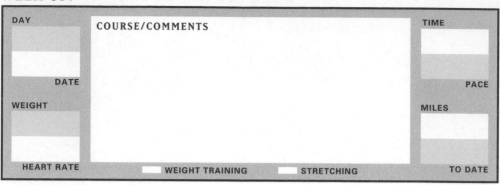

DAY

DATE

WEIGHT

HEART RATE

COURSE/COMMENTS

WEIGHT TRAINING STRETCHING

TIME

PACE

MILES

TO DATE

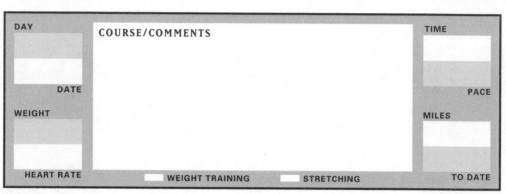

DAY

DATE

WEIGHT

HEART RATE

COURSE/COMMENTS

WEIGHT TRAINING STRETCHING

TIME

PACE

MILES

TO DATE

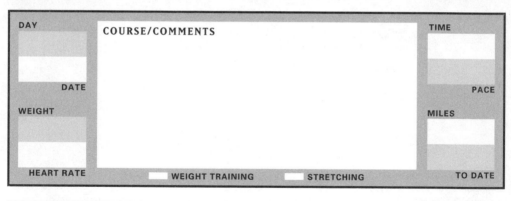

DAY

DATE

WEIGHT

HEART RATE

COURSE/COMMENTS

WEIGHT TRAINING STRETCHING

TIME

PACE

MILES

TO DATE

DAY

DATE

WEIGHT

HEART RATE

COURSE/COMMENTS

WEIGHT TRAINING STRETCHING

TIME

PACE

MILES

TO DATE

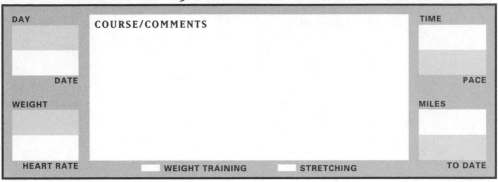

DAY

DATE

WEIGHT

HEART RATE

COURSE/COMMENTS

WEIGHT TRAINING   STRETCHING

TIME

PACE

MILES

TO DATE

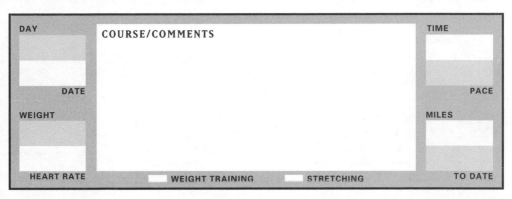

DAY

DATE

WEIGHT

HEART RATE

COURSE/COMMENTS

WEIGHT TRAINING   STRETCHING

TIME

PACE

MILES

TO DATE

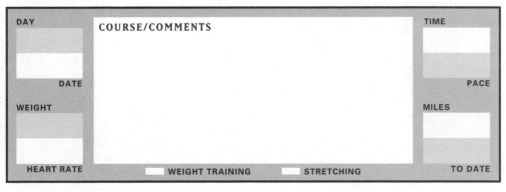

DAY

DATE

WEIGHT

HEART RATE

COURSE/COMMENTS

WEIGHT TRAINING   STRETCHING

TIME

PACE

MILES

TO DATE

WEEKLY SUMMARY
Longest Run _____
Total # Workouts
  Runs   _____
  Speed training _____
  Cross training _____
  Weight training_____
  Stretching   _____

WEEKLY TOTAL

YEAR TO DATE

WEEK OF:

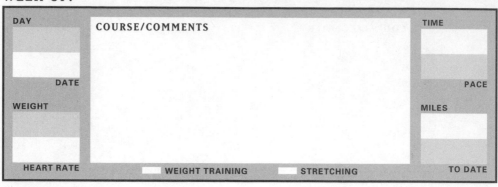

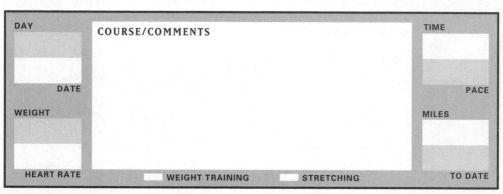

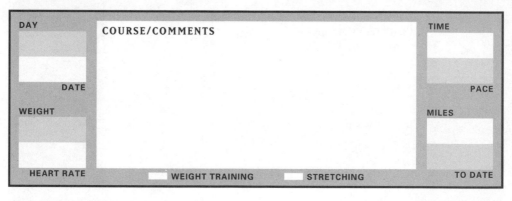

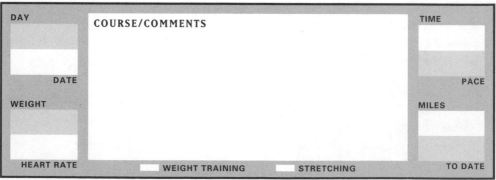

DAY

DATE

WEIGHT

HEART RATE

COURSE/COMMENTS

☐ WEIGHT TRAINING   ☐ STRETCHING

TIME

PACE

MILES

TO DATE

DAY

DATE

WEIGHT

HEART RATE

COURSE/COMMENTS

☐ WEIGHT TRAINING   ☐ STRETCHING

TIME

PACE

MILES

TO DATE

DAY

DATE

WEIGHT

HEART RATE

COURSE/COMMENTS

☐ WEIGHT TRAINING   ☐ STRETCHING

TIME

PACE

MILES

TO DATE

WEEKLY SUMMARY

Longest Run _____

Total # Workouts

Runs _____

Speed training _____

Cross training _____

Weight training_____

Stretching _____

WEEKLY TOTAL

YEAR TO DATE

WEEK OF:

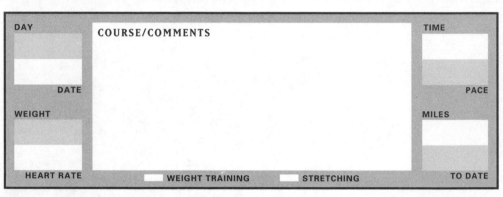

DAY

DATE

WEIGHT

HEART RATE

COURSE/COMMENTS

☐ **WEIGHT TRAINING** ☐ **STRETCHING**

TIME

PACE

MILES

TO DATE

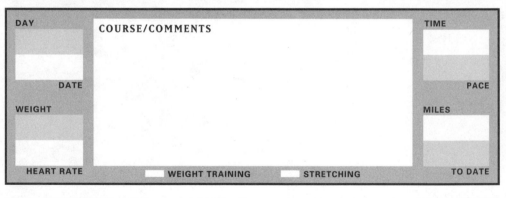

DAY

DATE

WEIGHT

HEART RATE

COURSE/COMMENTS

☐ **WEIGHT TRAINING** ☐ **STRETCHING**

TIME

PACE

MILES

TO DATE

DAY

DATE

WEIGHT

HEART RATE

COURSE/COMMENTS

☐ **WEIGHT TRAINING** ☐ **STRETCHING**

TIME

PACE

MILES

TO DATE

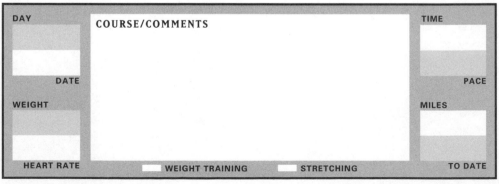

DAY

DATE

WEIGHT

HEART RATE

COURSE/COMMENTS

☐ **WEIGHT TRAINING** ☐ **STRETCHING**

TIME

PACE

MILES

TO DATE

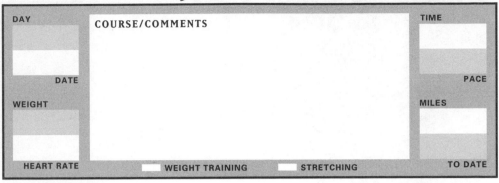

DAY

DATE

WEIGHT

HEART RATE

COURSE/COMMENTS

☐ WEIGHT TRAINING   ☐ STRETCHING

TIME

PACE

MILES

TO DATE

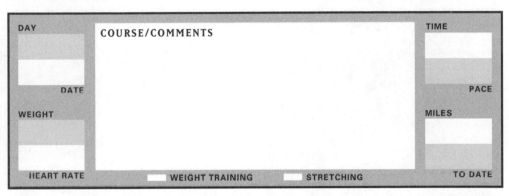

DAY

DATE

WEIGHT

HEART RATE

COURSE/COMMENTS

☐ WEIGHT TRAINING   ☐ STRETCHING

TIME

PACE

MILES

TO DATE

DAY

DATE

WEIGHT

HEART RATE

COURSE/COMMENTS

☐ WEIGHT TRAINING   ☐ STRETCHING

TIME

PACE

MILES

TO DATE

WEEKLY SUMMARY

Longest Run _____

Total # Workouts

Runs _____

Speed training _____

Cross training _____

Weight training _____

Stretching _____

WEEKLY TOTAL

YEAR TO DATE

WEEK OF:

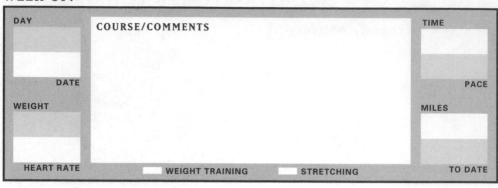

DAY

DATE

WEIGHT

HEART RATE

COURSE/COMMENTS

WEIGHT TRAINING   STRETCHING

TIME

PACE

MILES

TO DATE

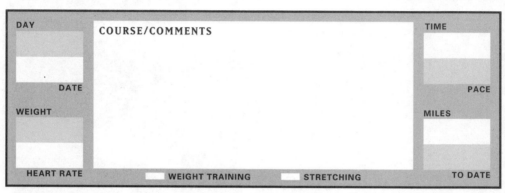

DAY

DATE

WEIGHT

HEART RATE

COURSE/COMMENTS

WEIGHT TRAINING   STRETCHING

TIME

PACE

MILES

TO DATE

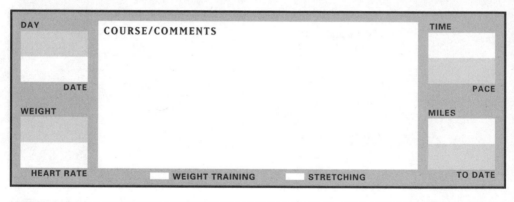

DAY

DATE

WEIGHT

HEART RATE

COURSE/COMMENTS

WEIGHT TRAINING   STRETCHING

TIME

PACE

MILES

TO DATE

DAY

DATE

WEIGHT

HEART RATE

COURSE/COMMENTS

WEIGHT TRAINING   STRETCHING

TIME

PACE

MILES

TO DATE

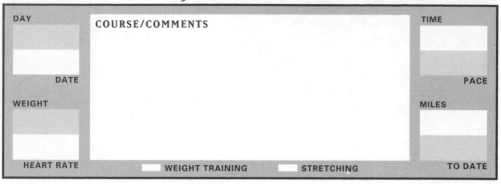

DAY

DATE

WEIGHT

HEART RATE

COURSE/COMMENTS

WEIGHT TRAINING   STRETCHING

TIME

PACE

MILES

TO DATE

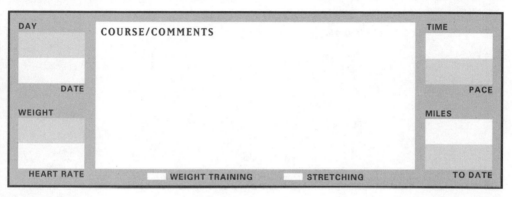

DAY

DATE

WEIGHT

HEART RATE

COURSE/COMMENTS

WEIGHT TRAINING   STRETCHING

TIME

PACE

MILES

TO DATE

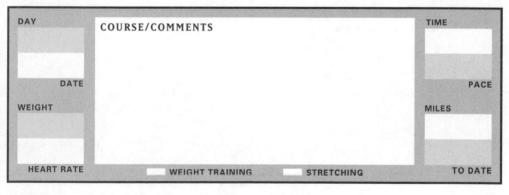

DAY

DATE

WEIGHT

HEART RATE

COURSE/COMMENTS

WEIGHT TRAINING   STRETCHING

TIME

PACE

MILES

TO DATE

WEEKLY SUMMARY

Longest Run _____

Total # Workouts

Runs _____

Speed training _____

Cross training _____

Weight training _____

Stretching _____

WEEKLY TOTAL

YEAR TO DATE

WEEK OF:

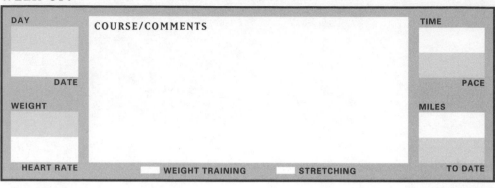

DAY

DATE

WEIGHT

HEART RATE

COURSE/COMMENTS

☐ WEIGHT TRAINING   ☐ STRETCHING

TIME

PACE

MILES

TO DATE

DAY

DATE

WEIGHT

HEART RATE

COURSE/COMMENTS

☐ WEIGHT TRAINING   ☐ STRETCHING

TIME

PACE

MILES

TO DATE

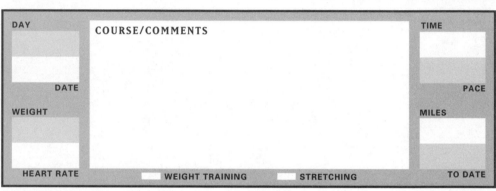

DAY

DATE

WEIGHT

HEART RATE

COURSE/COMMENTS

☐ WEIGHT TRAINING   ☐ STRETCHING

TIME

PACE

MILES

TO DATE

DAY

DATE

WEIGHT

HEART RATE

COURSE/COMMENTS

☐ WEIGHT TRAINING   ☐ STRETCHING

TIME

PACE

MILES

TO DATE

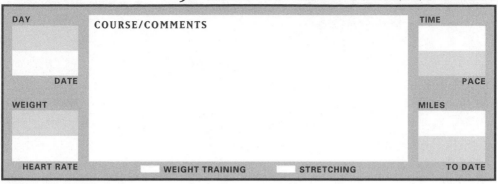

DAY	COURSE/COMMENTS	TIME
DATE		PACE
WEIGHT		MILES
HEART RATE	WEIGHT TRAINING STRETCHING	TO DATE

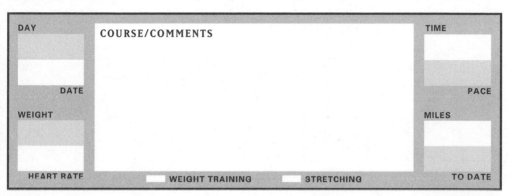

DAY	COURSE/COMMENTS	TIME
DATE		PACE
WEIGHT		MILES
HEART RATE	WEIGHT TRAINING STRETCHING	TO DATE

DAY	COURSE/COMMENTS	TIME
DATE		PACE
WEIGHT		MILES
HEART RATE	WEIGHT TRAINING STRETCHING	TO DATE

WEEKLY SUMMARY

Longest Run _____

Total # Workouts

Runs _____

Speed training _____

Cross training _____

Weight training_____

Stretching _____

WEEKLY TOTAL

YEAR TO DATE

WEEK OF:

DAY

DATE

WEIGHT

HEART RATE

COURSE/COMMENTS

☐ WEIGHT TRAINING   ☐ STRETCHING

TIME

PACE

MILES

TO DATE

DAY

DATE

WEIGHT

HEART RATE

COURSE/COMMENTS

☐ WEIGHT TRAINING   ☐ STRETCHING

TIME

PACE

MILES

TO DATE

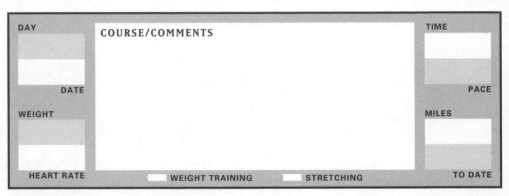

DAY

DATE

WEIGHT

HEART RATE

COURSE/COMMENTS

☐ WEIGHT TRAINING   ☐ STRETCHING

TIME

PACE

MILES

TO DATE

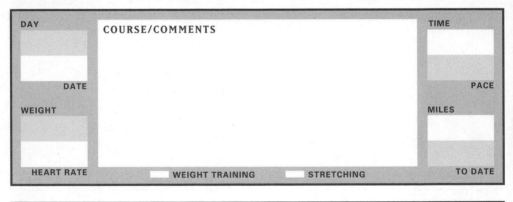

DAY

DATE

WEIGHT

HEART RATE

COURSE/COMMENTS

☐ WEIGHT TRAINING   ☐ STRETCHING

TIME

PACE

MILES

TO DATE

84

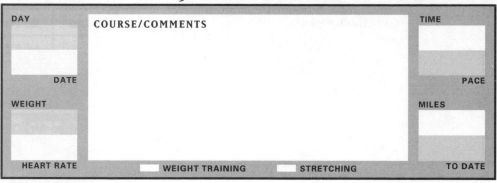

DAY	COURSE/COMMENTS	TIME
DATE		PACE
WEIGHT		MILES
HEART RATE	WEIGHT TRAINING STRETCHING	TO DATE

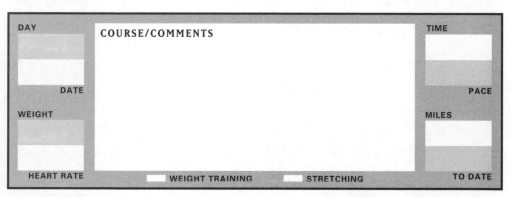

DAY	COURSE/COMMENTS	TIME
DATE		PACE
WEIGHT		MILES
HEART RATE	WEIGHT TRAINING STRETCHING	TO DATE

DAY	COURSE/COMMENTS	TIME
DATE		PACE
WEIGHT		MILES
HEART RATE	WEIGHT TRAINING STRETCHING	TO DATE

WEEKLY SUMMARY

Longest Run _____

Total # Workouts

Runs _____

Speed training _____

Cross training _____

Weight training _____

Stretching _____

WEEKLY TOTAL

YEAR TO DATE

WEEK OF:

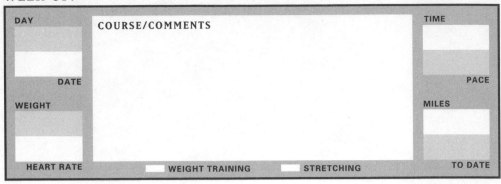

DAY

DATE

WEIGHT

HEART RATE

COURSE/COMMENTS

WEIGHT TRAINING   STRETCHING

TIME

PACE

MILES

TO DATE

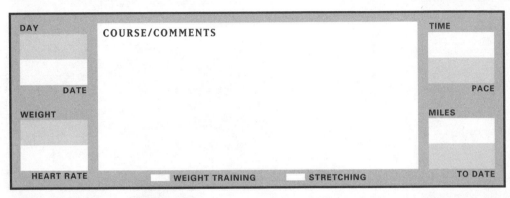

DAY

DATE

WEIGHT

HEART RATE

COURSE/COMMENTS

WEIGHT TRAINING   STRETCHING

TIME

PACE

MILES

TO DATE

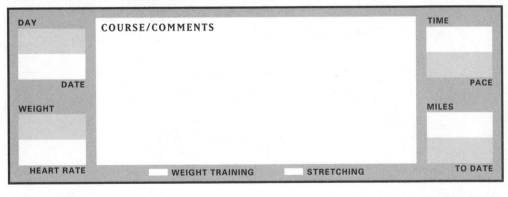

DAY

DATE

WEIGHT

HEART RATE

COURSE/COMMENTS

WEIGHT TRAINING   STRETCHING

TIME

PACE

MILES

TO DATE

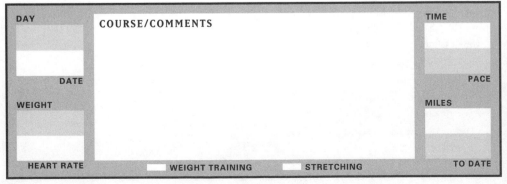

DAY

DATE

WEIGHT

HEART RATE

COURSE/COMMENTS

WEIGHT TRAINING   STRETCHING

TIME

PACE

MILES

TO DATE

DAY

COURSE/COMMENTS

TIME

DATE

PACE

WEIGHT

MILES

HEART RATE   WEIGHT TRAINING   STRETCHING   TO DATE

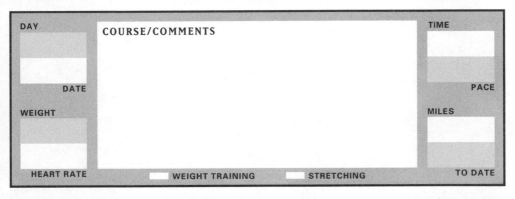

DAY

COURSE/COMMENTS

TIME

DATE

PACE

WEIGHT

MILES

HEART RATE   WEIGHT TRAINING   STRETCHING   TO DATE

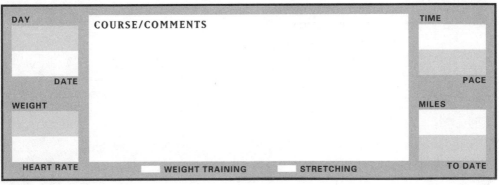

DAY

COURSE/COMMENTS

TIME

DATE

PACE

WEIGHT

MILES

HEART RATE   WEIGHT TRAINING   STRETCHING   TO DATE

WEEKLY SUMMARY

Longest Run _____

Total # Workouts

Runs _____

Speed training _____

Cross training _____

Weight training _____

Stretching _____

WEEKLY TOTAL

YEAR TO DATE

WEEK OF:

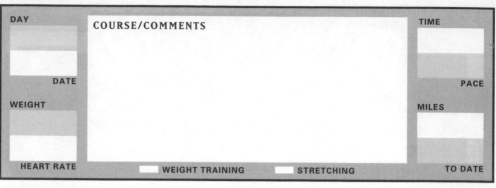

DAY

COURSE/COMMENTS

TIME

DATE

PACE

WEIGHT

MILES

HEART RATE   WEIGHT TRAINING   STRETCHING   TO DATE

DAY

COURSE/COMMENTS

TIME

DATE

PACE

WEIGHT

MILES

HEART RATE   WEIGHT TRAINING   STRETCHING   TO DATE

DAY

COURSE/COMMENTS

TIME

DATE

PACE

WEIGHT

MILES

HEART RATE   WEIGHT TRAINING   STRETCHING   TO DATE

DAY

COURSE/COMMENTS

TIME

DATE

PACE

WEIGHT

MILES

HEART RATE   WEIGHT TRAINING   STRETCHING   TO DATE

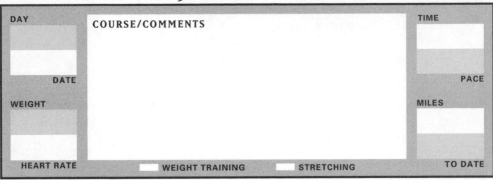

DAY

DATE

WEIGHT

HEART RATE

COURSE/COMMENTS

WEIGHT TRAINING ☐ STRETCHING ☐

TIME

PACE

MILES

TO DATE

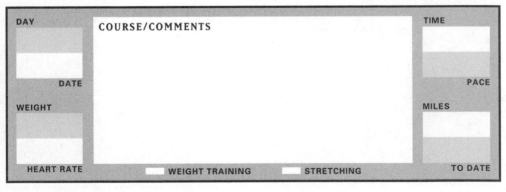

DAY

DATE

WEIGHT

HEART RATE

COURSE/COMMENTS

WEIGHT TRAINING ☐ STRETCHING ☐

TIME

PACE

MILES

TO DATE

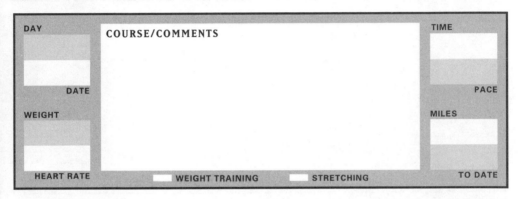

DAY

DATE

WEIGHT

HEART RATE

COURSE/COMMENTS

WEIGHT TRAINING ☐ STRETCHING ☐

TIME

PACE

MILES

TO DATE

WEEKLY SUMMARY

Longest Run _____

Total # Workouts

Runs _____

Speed training _____

Cross training _____

Weight training _____

Stretching _____

WEEKLY TOTAL

YEAR TO DATE

WEEK OF:

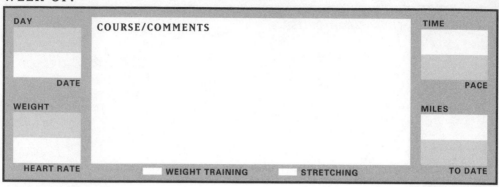

DAY

DATE

WEIGHT

HEART RATE

COURSE/COMMENTS

□ WEIGHT TRAINING   □ STRETCHING

TIME

PACE

MILES

TO DATE

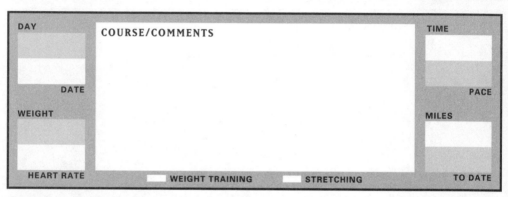

DAY

DATE

WEIGHT

HEART RATE

COURSE/COMMENTS

□ WEIGHT TRAINING   □ STRETCHING

TIME

PACE

MILES

TO DATE

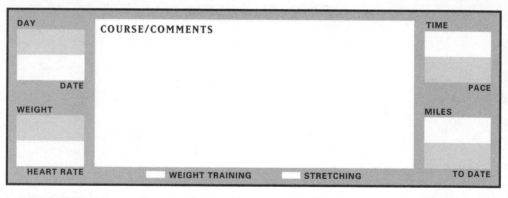

DAY

DATE

WEIGHT

HEART RATE

COURSE/COMMENTS

□ WEIGHT TRAINING   □ STRETCHING

TIME

PACE

MILES

TO DATE

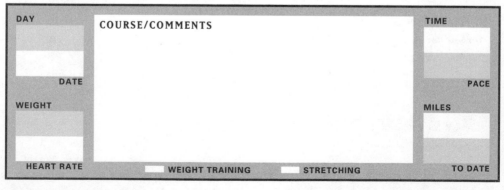

DAY

DATE

WEIGHT

HEART RATE

COURSE/COMMENTS

□ WEIGHT TRAINING   □ STRETCHING

TIME

PACE

MILES

TO DATE

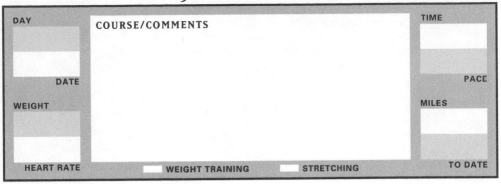

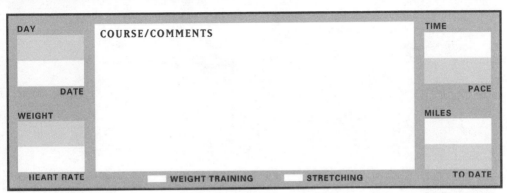

DAY	COURSE/COMMENTS	TIME
DATE		PACE
WEIGHT		MILES
HEART RATE	WEIGHT TRAINING STRETCHING	TO DATE

WEEKLY SUMMARY

Longest Run _____

Total # Workouts

Runs _____

Speed training _____

Cross training _____

Weight training _____

Stretching _____

WEEKLY TOTAL

YEAR TO DATE

WEEK OF:

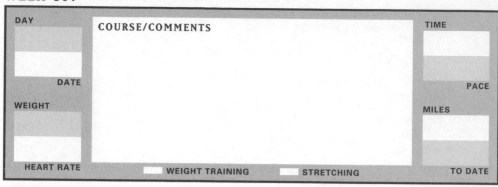

DAY

DATE

WEIGHT

HEART RATE

COURSE/COMMENTS

WEIGHT TRAINING · STRETCHING

TIME

PACE

MILES

TO DATE

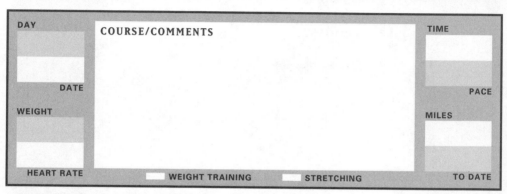

DAY

DATE

WEIGHT

HEART RATE

COURSE/COMMENTS

WEIGHT TRAINING · STRETCHING

TIME

PACE

MILES

TO DATE

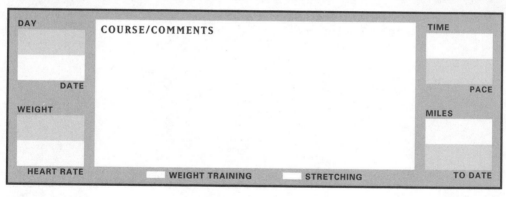

DAY

DATE

WEIGHT

HEART RATE

COURSE/COMMENTS

WEIGHT TRAINING · STRETCHING

TIME

PACE

MILES

TO DATE

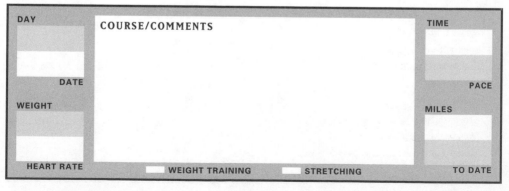

DAY

DATE

WEIGHT

HEART RATE

COURSE/COMMENTS

WEIGHT TRAINING · STRETCHING

TIME

PACE

MILES

TO DATE

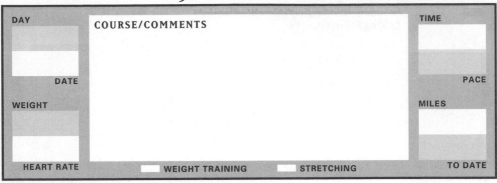

DAY	COURSE/COMMENTS	TIME
DATE		PACE
WEIGHT		MILES
HEART RATE	WEIGHT TRAINING ☐ STRETCHING ☐	TO DATE

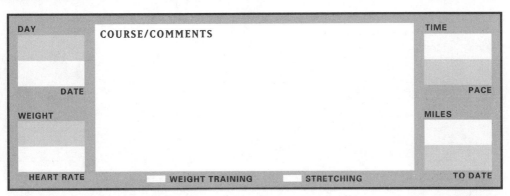

DAY	COURSE/COMMENTS	TIME
DATE		PACE
WEIGHT		MILES
HEART RATE	WEIGHT TRAINING ☐ STRETCHING ☐	TO DATE

DAY	COURSE/COMMENTS	TIME
DATE		PACE
WEIGHT		MILES
HEART RATE	WEIGHT TRAINING ☐ STRETCHING ☐	TO DATE

WEEKLY SUMMARY

Longest Run _____

Total # Workouts

Runs _____

Speed training _____

Cross training _____

Weight training_____

Stretching _____

WEEKLY TOTAL

YEAR TO DATE

WEEK OF:

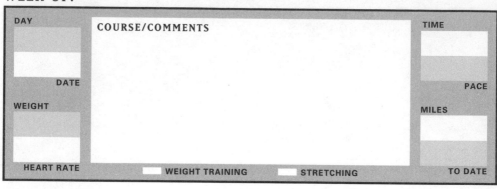

DAY

DATE

WEIGHT

HEART RATE

COURSE/COMMENTS

WEIGHT TRAINING   STRETCHING

TIME

PACE

MILES

TO DATE

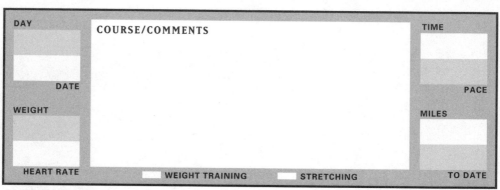

DAY

DATE

WEIGHT

HEART RATE

COURSE/COMMENTS

WEIGHT TRAINING   STRETCHING

TIME

PACE

MILES

TO DATE

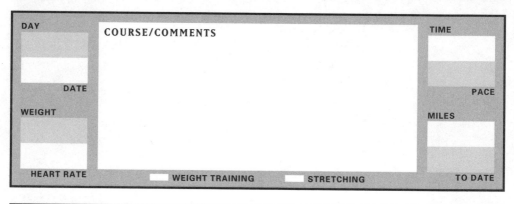

DAY

DATE

WEIGHT

HEART RATE

COURSE/COMMENTS

WEIGHT TRAINING   STRETCHING

TIME

PACE

MILES

TO DATE

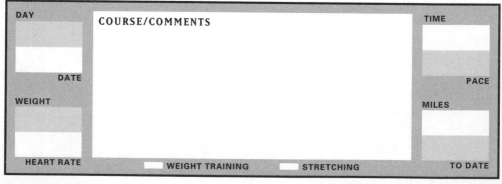

DAY

DATE

WEIGHT

HEART RATE

COURSE/COMMENTS

WEIGHT TRAINING   STRETCHING

TIME

PACE

MILES

TO DATE

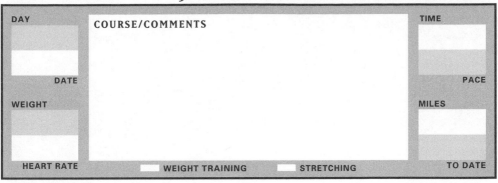

DAY

DATE

WEIGHT

HEART RATE

COURSE/COMMENTS

WEIGHT TRAINING   STRETCHING

TIME

PACE

MILES

TO DATE

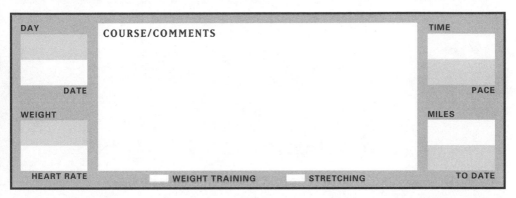

DAY

DATE

WEIGHT

HEART RATE

COURSE/COMMENTS

WEIGHT TRAINING   STRETCHING

TIME

PACE

MILES

TO DATE

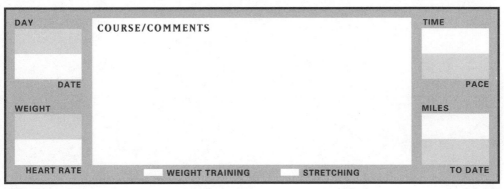

DAY

DATE

WEIGHT

HEART RATE

COURSE/COMMENTS

WEIGHT TRAINING   STRETCHING

TIME

PACE

MILES

TO DATE

WEEKLY SUMMARY

Longest Run _____

Total # Workouts

  Runs   _____

  Speed training _____

  Cross training _____

  Weight training _____

  Stretching   _____

WEEKLY TOTAL

YEAR TO DATE

WEEK OF:

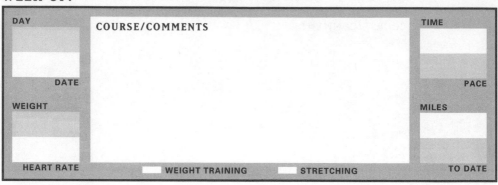

DAY

DATE

WEIGHT

HEART RATE

COURSE/COMMENTS

◻ WEIGHT TRAINING   ◻ STRETCHING

TIME

PACE

MILES

TO DATE

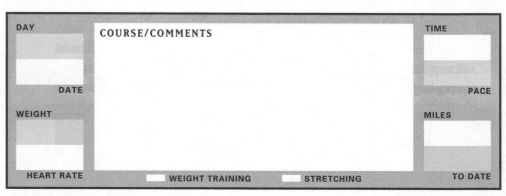

DAY

DATE

WEIGHT

HEART RATE

COURSE/COMMENTS

◻ WEIGHT TRAINING   ◻ STRETCHING

TIME

PACE

MILES

TO DATE

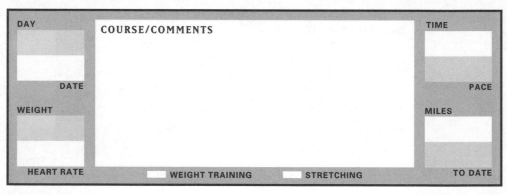

DAY

DATE

WEIGHT

HEART RATE

COURSE/COMMENTS

◻ WEIGHT TRAINING   ◻ STRETCHING

TIME

PACE

MILES

TO DATE

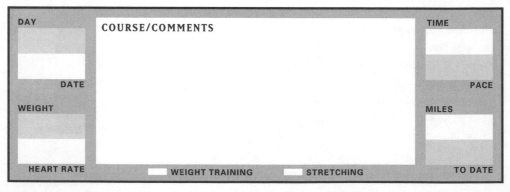

DAY

DATE

WEIGHT

HEART RATE

COURSE/COMMENTS

◻ WEIGHT TRAINING   ◻ STRETCHING

TIME

PACE

MILES

TO DATE

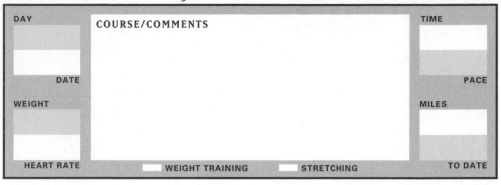

DAY	COURSE/COMMENTS	TIME
DATE		PACE
WEIGHT		MILES
HEART RATE	WEIGHT TRAINING STRETCHING	TO DATE

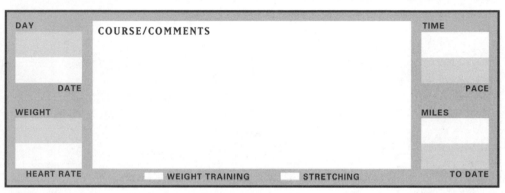

DAY	COURSE/COMMENTS	TIME
DATE		PACE
WEIGHT		MILES
HEART RATE	WEIGHT TRAINING STRETCHING	TO DATE

DAY	COURSE/COMMENTS	TIME
DATE		PACE
WEIGHT		MILES
HEART RATE	WEIGHT TRAINING STRETCHING	TO DATE

WEEKLY SUMMARY

Longest Run _____

Total # Workouts

Runs _____

Speed training _____

Cross training _____

Weight training_____

Stretching _____

WEEKLY TOTAL

YEAR TO DATE

WEEK OF:

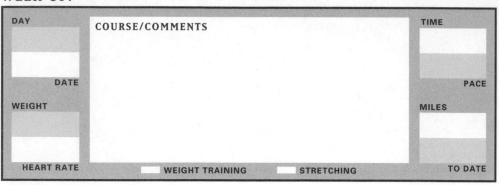

DAY

DATE

WEIGHT

HEART RATE

COURSE/COMMENTS

WEIGHT TRAINING   STRETCHING

TIME

PACE

MILES

TO DATE

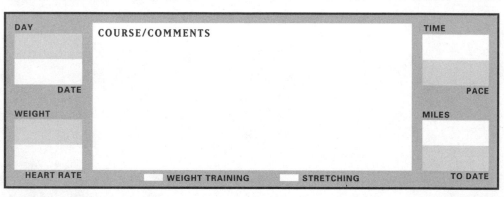

DAY

DATE

WEIGHT

HEART RATE

COURSE/COMMENTS

WEIGHT TRAINING   STRETCHING

TIME

PACE

MILES

TO DATE

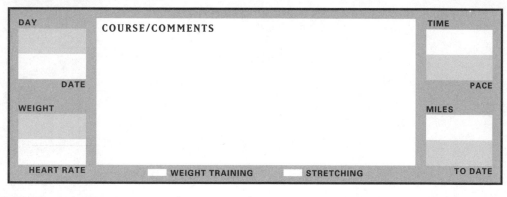

DAY

DATE

WEIGHT

HEART RATE

COURSE/COMMENTS

WEIGHT TRAINING   STRETCHING

TIME

PACE

MILES

TO DATE

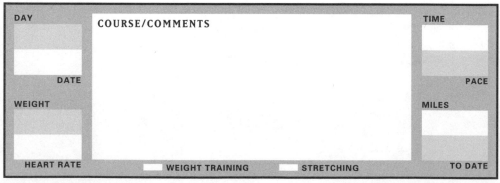

DAY

DATE

WEIGHT

HEART RATE

COURSE/COMMENTS

WEIGHT TRAINING   STRETCHING

TIME

PACE

MILES

TO DATE

DAY	COURSE/COMMENTS	TIME
DATE		PACE
WEIGHT		MILES
HEART RATE	WEIGHT TRAINING STRETCHING	TO DATE

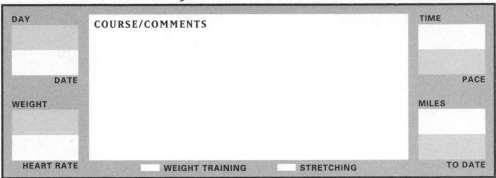

DAY	COURSE/COMMENTS	TIME
DATE		PACE
WEIGHT		MILES
HEART RATE	WEIGHT TRAINING STRETCHING	TO DATE

DAY	COURSE/COMMENTS	TIME
DATE		PACE
WEIGHT		MILES
HEART RATE	WEIGHT TRAINING STRETCHING	TO DATE

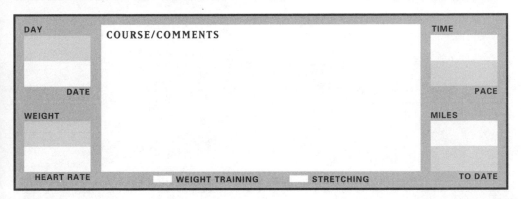

WEEKLY SUMMARY

Longest Run _____

Total # Workouts

Runs _____

Speed training _____

Cross training _____

Weight training _____

Stretching _____

WEEKLY TOTAL

YEAR TO DATE

WEEK OF:

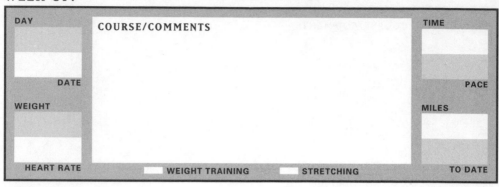

DAY

DATE

WEIGHT

HEART RATE

COURSE/COMMENTS

☐ WEIGHT TRAINING   ☐ STRETCHING

TIME

PACE

MILES

TO DATE

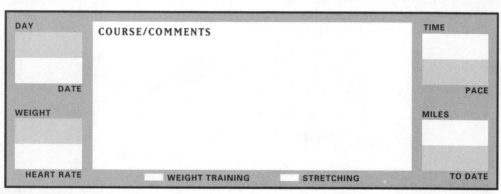

DAY

DATE

WEIGHT

HEART RATE

COURSE/COMMENTS

☐ WEIGHT TRAINING   ☐ STRETCHING

TIME

PACE

MILES

TO DATE

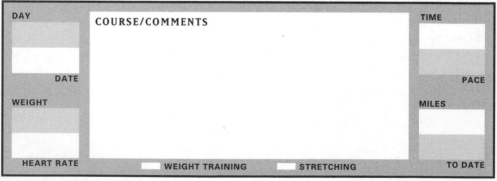

DAY

DATE

WEIGHT

HEART RATE

COURSE/COMMENTS

☐ WEIGHT TRAINING   ☐ STRETCHING

TIME

PACE

MILES

TO DATE

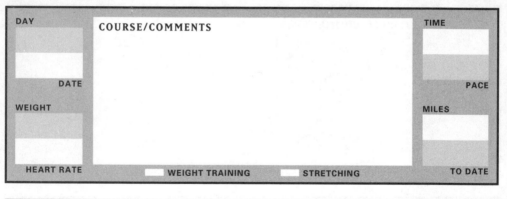

DAY

DATE

WEIGHT

HEART RATE

COURSE/COMMENTS

☐ WEIGHT TRAINING   ☐ STRETCHING

TIME

PACE

MILES

TO DATE

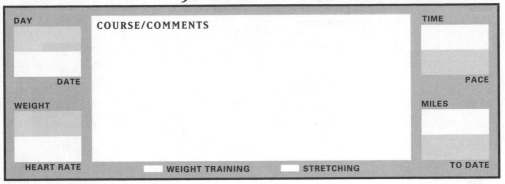

DAY

DATE

WEIGHT

HEART RATE

COURSE/COMMENTS

WEIGHT TRAINING   STRETCHING

TIME

PACE

MILES

TO DATE

DAY

DATE

WEIGHT

HEART RATE

COURSE/COMMENTS

WEIGHT TRAINING   STRETCHING

TIME

PACE

MILES

TO DATE

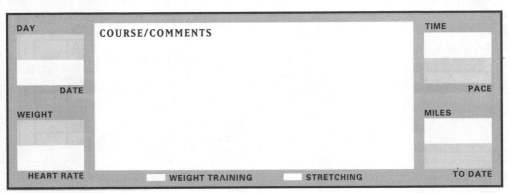

DAY

DATE

WEIGHT

HEART RATE

COURSE/COMMENTS

WEIGHT TRAINING   STRETCHING

TIME

PACE

MILES

TO DATE

WEEKLY SUMMARY

Longest Run _____

Total # Workouts

Runs _____

Speed training _____

Cross training _____

Weight training _____

Stretching _____

WEEKLY TOTAL

YEAR TO DATE

WEEK OF:

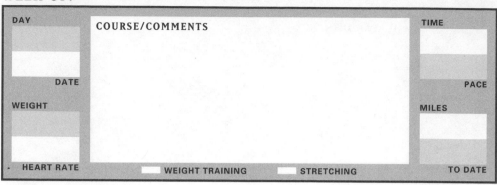

DAY

DATE

WEIGHT

HEART RATE

COURSE/COMMENTS

⬜ WEIGHT TRAINING   ⬜ STRETCHING

TIME

PACE

MILES

TO DATE

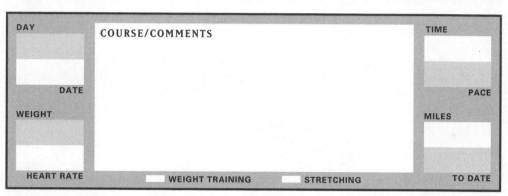

DAY

DATE

WEIGHT

HEART RATE

COURSE/COMMENTS

⬜ WEIGHT TRAINING   ⬜ STRETCHING

TIME

PACE

MILES

TO DATE

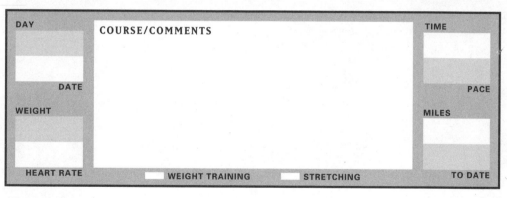

DAY

DATE

WEIGHT

HEART RATE

COURSE/COMMENTS

⬜ WEIGHT TRAINING   ⬜ STRETCHING

TIME

PACE

MILES

TO DATE

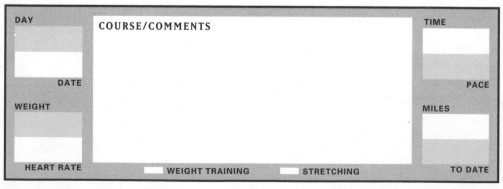

DAY

DATE

WEIGHT

HEART RATE

COURSE/COMMENTS

⬜ WEIGHT TRAINING   ⬜ STRETCHING

TIME

PACE

MILES

TO DATE

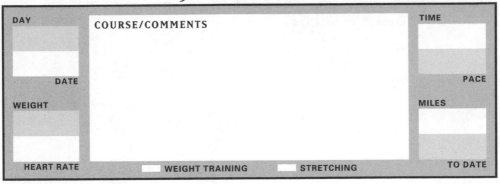

DAY	COURSE/COMMENTS		TIME
DATE			PACE
WEIGHT			MILES
HEART RATE	☐ WEIGHT TRAINING ☐ STRETCHING		TO DATE

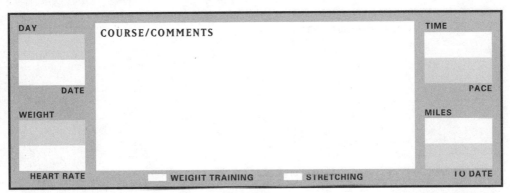

DAY	COURSE/COMMENTS		TIME
DATE			PACE
WEIGHT			MILES
HEART RATE	☐ WEIGHT TRAINING ☐ STRETCHING		TO DATE

DAY	COURSE/COMMENTS		TIME
DATE			PACE
WEIGHT			MILES
HEART RATE	☐ WEIGHT TRAINING ☐ STRETCHING		TO DATE

WEEKLY SUMMARY

Longest Run _____

Total # Workouts

Runs _____

Speed training _____

Cross training _____

Weight training _____

Stretching _____

WEEKLY TOTAL

YEAR TO DATE

WEEK OF:

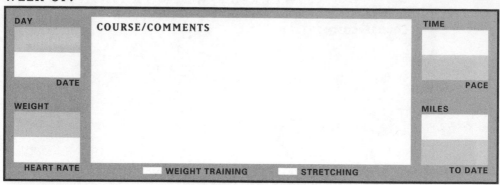

DAY

DATE

WEIGHT

HEART RATE

COURSE/COMMENTS

☐ WEIGHT TRAINING ☐ STRETCHING

TIME

PACE

MILES

TO DATE

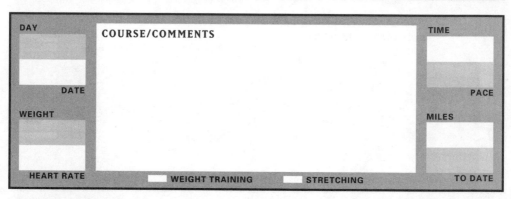

DAY

DATE

WEIGHT

HEART RATE

COURSE/COMMENTS

☐ WEIGHT TRAINING ☐ STRETCHING

TIME

PACE

MILES

TO DATE

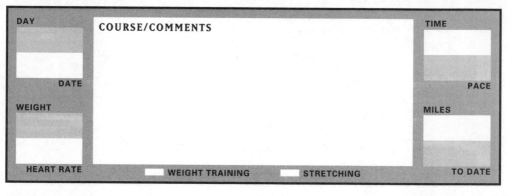

DAY

DATE

WEIGHT

HEART RATE

COURSE/COMMENTS

☐ WEIGHT TRAINING ☐ STRETCHING

TIME

PACE

MILES

TO DATE

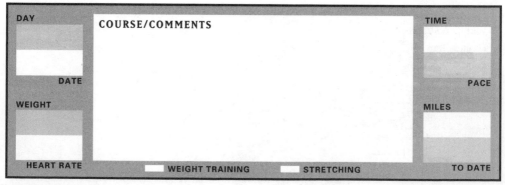

DAY

DATE

WEIGHT

HEART RATE

COURSE/COMMENTS

☐ WEIGHT TRAINING ☐ STRETCHING

TIME

PACE

MILES

TO DATE

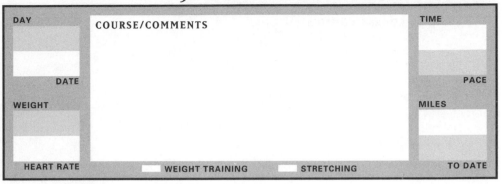

DAY

DATE

WEIGHT

HEART RATE

COURSE/COMMENTS

WEIGHT TRAINING   STRETCHING

TIME

PACE

MILES

TO DATE

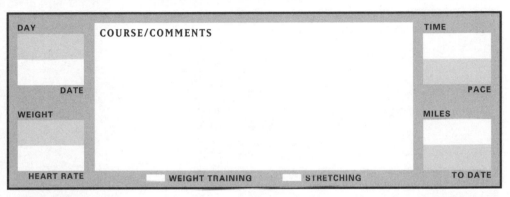

DAY

DATE

WEIGHT

HEART RATE

COURSE/COMMENTS

WEIGHT TRAINING   STRETCHING

TIME

PACE

MILES

TO DATE

DAY

DATE

WEIGHT

HEART RATE

COURSE/COMMENTS

WEIGHT TRAINING   STRETCHING

TIME

PACE

MILES

TO DATE

WEEKLY SUMMARY

Longest Run ⎯⎯⎯⎯

Total # Workouts

Runs ⎯⎯⎯⎯

Speed training ⎯⎯⎯⎯

Cross training ⎯⎯⎯⎯

Weight training ⎯⎯⎯⎯

Stretching ⎯⎯⎯⎯

WEEKLY TOTAL

YEAR TO DATE

WEEK OF:

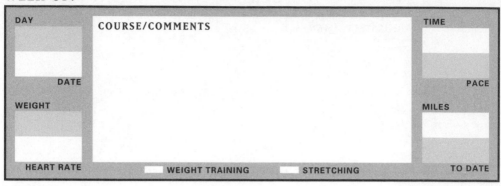

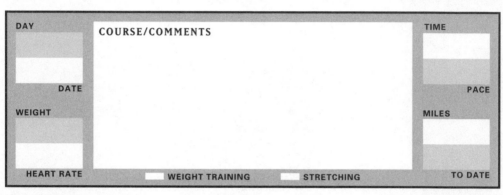

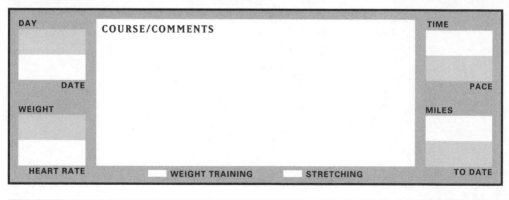

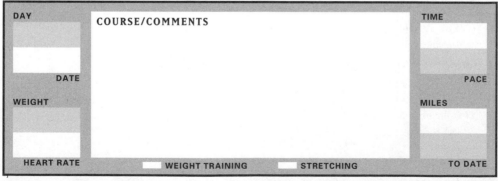

106

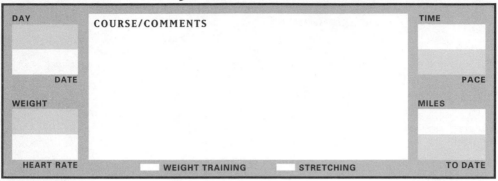

DAY

COURSE/COMMENTS

TIME

DATE

PACE

WEIGHT

MILES

HEART RATE　　WEIGHT TRAINING　　STRETCHING　　TO DATE

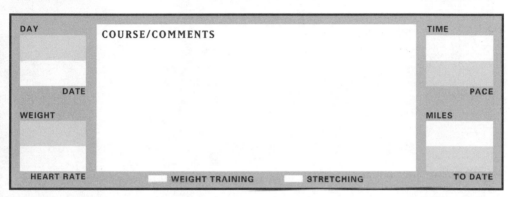

DAY

COURSE/COMMENTS

TIME

DATE

PACE

WEIGHT

MILES

HEART RATE　　WEIGHT TRAINING　　STRETCHING　　TO DATE

DAY

COURSE/COMMENTS

TIME

DATE

PACE

WEIGHT

MILES

HEART RATE　　WEIGHT TRAINING　　STRETCHING　　TO DATE

WEEKLY SUMMARY
Longest Run _____
Total # Workouts
　Runs　　　　　_____
　Speed training _____
　Cross training _____
　Weight training_____
　Stretching　　_____

WEEKLY TOTAL

YEAR TO DATE

WEEK OF:

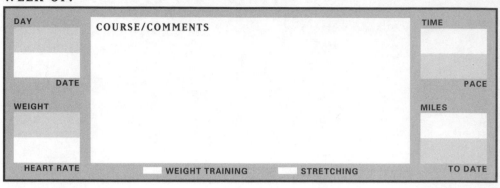

DAY

DATE

WEIGHT

HEART RATE

COURSE/COMMENTS

☐ WEIGHT TRAINING   ☐ STRETCHING

TIME

PACE

MILES

TO DATE

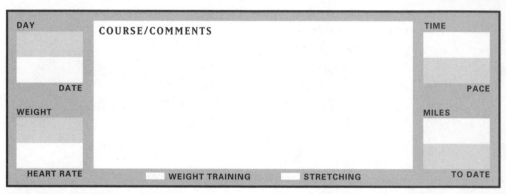

DAY

DATE

WEIGHT

HEART RATE

COURSE/COMMENTS

☐ WEIGHT TRAINING   ☐ STRETCHING

TIME

PACE

MILES

TO DATE

DAY

DATE

WEIGHT

HEART RATE

COURSE/COMMENTS

☐ WEIGHT TRAINING   ☐ STRETCHING

TIME

PACE

MILES

TO DATE

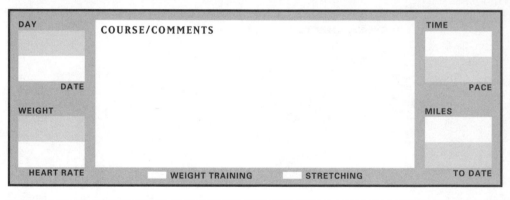

DAY

DATE

WEIGHT

HEART RATE

COURSE/COMMENTS

☐ WEIGHT TRAINING   ☐ STRETCHING

TIME

PACE

MILES

TO DATE

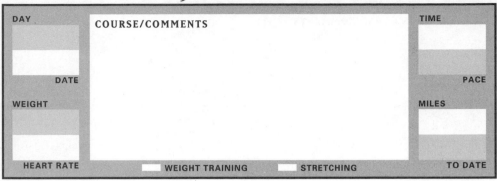

DAY

DATE

WEIGHT

HEART RATE

COURSE/COMMENTS

WEIGHT TRAINING   STRETCHING

TIME

PACE

MILES

TO DATE

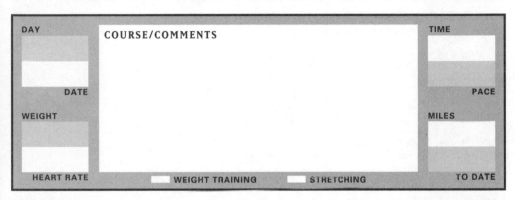

DAY

DATE

WEIGHT

HEART RATE

COURSE/COMMENTS

WEIGHT TRAINING   STRETCHING

TIME

PACE

MILES

TO DATE

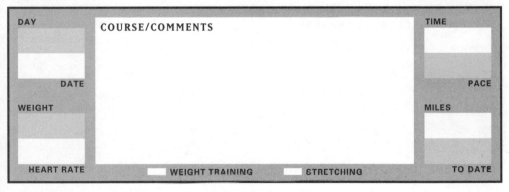

DAY

DATE

WEIGHT

HEART RATE

COURSE/COMMENTS

WEIGHT TRAINING   STRETCHING

TIME

PACE

MILES

TO DATE

WEEKLY SUMMARY

Longest Run _____

Total # Workouts

Runs _____

Speed training _____

Cross training _____

Weight training _____

Stretching _____

WEEKLY TOTAL

YEAR TO DATE

WEEK OF:

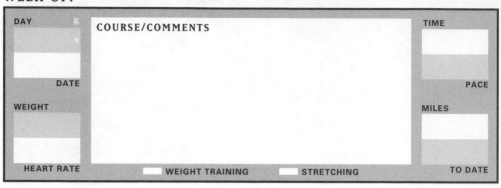

DAY

DATE

WEIGHT

HEART RATE

COURSE/COMMENTS

☐ WEIGHT TRAINING   ☐ STRETCHING

TIME

PACE

MILES

TO DATE

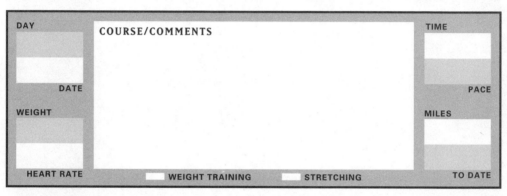

DAY

DATE

WEIGHT

HEART RATE

COURSE/COMMENTS

☐ WEIGHT TRAINING   ☐ STRETCHING

TIME

PACE

MILES

TO DATE

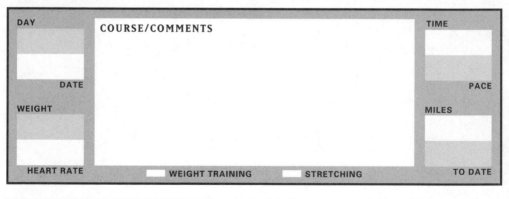

DAY

DATE

WEIGHT

HEART RATE

COURSE/COMMENTS

☐ WEIGHT TRAINING   ☐ STRETCHING

TIME

PACE

MILES

TO DATE

DAY

DATE

WEIGHT

HEART RATE

COURSE/COMMENTS

☐ WEIGHT TRAINING   ☐ STRETCHING

TIME

PACE

MILES

TO DATE

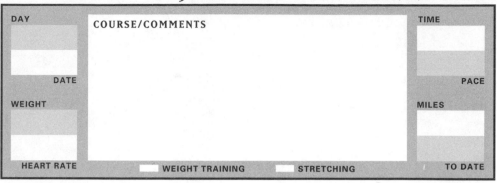

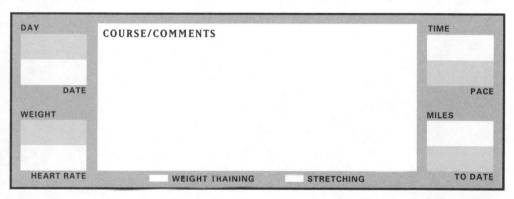

DAY

DATE

WEIGHT

HEART RATE

COURSE/COMMENTS

WEIGHT TRAINING

STRETCHING

TIME

PACE

MILES

TO DATE

WEEKLY SUMMARY

Longest Run _____

Total # Workouts

  Runs _____

  Speed training _____

  Cross training _____

  Weight training _____

  Stretching _____

WEEKLY TOTAL

YEAR TO DATE

WEEK OF:

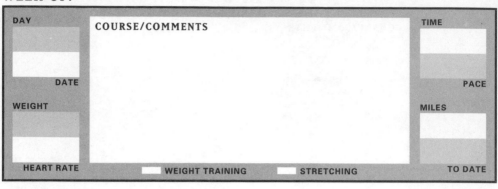

DAY

DATE

WEIGHT

HEART RATE

COURSE/COMMENTS

☐ WEIGHT TRAINING   ☐ STRETCHING

TIME

PACE

MILES

TO DATE

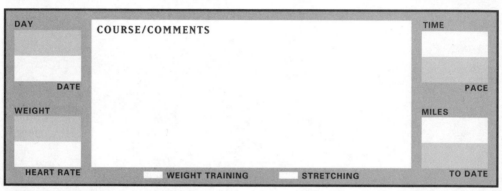

DAY

DATE

WEIGHT

HEART RATE

COURSE/COMMENTS

☐ WEIGHT TRAINING   ☐ STRETCHING

TIME

PACE

MILES

TO DATE

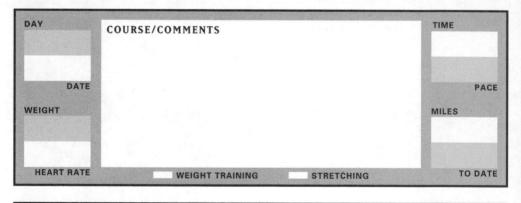

DAY

DATE

WEIGHT

HEART RATE

COURSE/COMMENTS

☐ WEIGHT TRAINING   ☐ STRETCHING

TIME

PACE

MILES

TO DATE

DAY

DATE

WEIGHT

HEART RATE

COURSE/COMMENTS

☐ WEIGHT TRAINING   ☐ STRETCHING

TIME

PACE

MILES

TO DATE

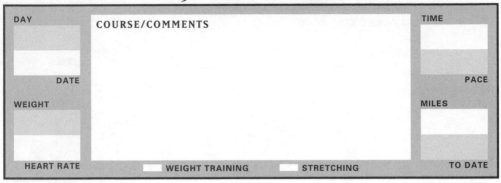

DAY	COURSE/COMMENTS	TIME
DATE		PACE
WEIGHT		MILES
HEART RATE	WEIGHT TRAINING STRETCHING	TO DATE

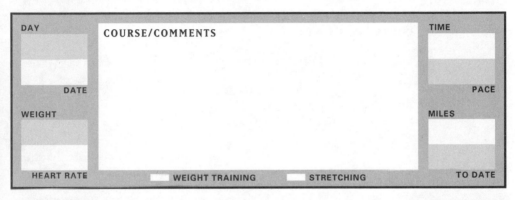

DAY	COURSE/COMMENTS	TIME
DATE		PACE
WEIGHT		MILES
HEART RATE	WEIGHT TRAINING STRETCHING	TO DATE

DAY	COURSE/COMMENTS	TIME
DATE		PACE
WEIGHT		MILES
HEART RATE	WEIGHT TRAINING STRETCHING	TO DATE

WEEKLY SUMMARY

Longest Run _____

Total # Workouts

Runs _____

Speed training _____

Cross training _____

Weight training _____

Stretching _____

WEEKLY TOTAL

YEAR TO DATE

WEEK OF:

DAY

DATE

WEIGHT

HEART RATE

COURSE/COMMENTS

☐ **WEIGHT TRAINING**   ☐ **STRETCHING**

TIME

PACE

MILES

TO DATE

DAY

DATE

WEIGHT

HEART RATE

COURSE/COMMENTS

☐ **WEIGHT TRAINING**   ☐ **STRETCHING**

TIME

PACE

MILES

TO DATE

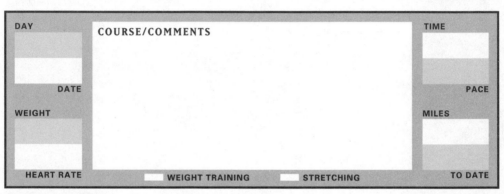

DAY

DATE

WEIGHT

HEART RATE

COURSE/COMMENTS

☐ **WEIGHT TRAINING**   ☐ **STRETCHING**

TIME

PACE

MILES

TO DATE

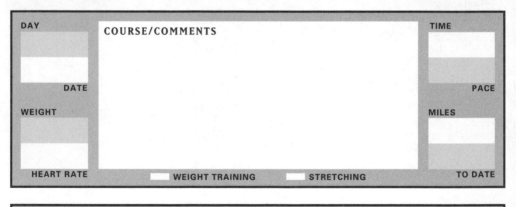

DAY

DATE

WEIGHT

HEART RATE

COURSE/COMMENTS

☐ **WEIGHT TRAINING**   ☐ **STRETCHING**

TIME

PACE

MILES

TO DATE

DAY

DATE

WEIGHT

HEART RATE

COURSE/COMMENTS

☐ WEIGHT TRAINING   ☐ STRETCHING

TIME

PACE

MILES

TO DATE

DAY

DATE

WEIGHT

HFART RATE

COURSE/COMMENTS

☐ WEIGHT TRAINING   ☐ STRETCHING

TIME

PACE

MILES

TO DATE

DAY

DATE

WEIGHT

HEART RATE

COURSE/COMMENTS

☐ WEIGHT TRAINING   ☐ STRETCHING

TIME

PACE

MILES

TO DATE

WEEKLY SUMMARY

Longest Run _____

Total # Workouts

Runs _____

Speed training _____

Cross training _____

Weight training_____

Stretching _____

WEEKLY TOTAL

YEAR TO DATE

WEEK-BY-WEEK MILEAGE CHART			
WEEK	DATE	MILEAGE	COMMENTS
1			
2			
3			
4			
5			
6			
7			
8			
9			
10			
11			
12			
13			
14			
15			
16			
17			
18			
19			
20			
21			
22			
23			
24			
25			
26			

WEEK	DATE	MILEAGE	COMMENTS
27			
28			
29			
30			
31			
32			
33			
34			
35			
36			
37			
38			
39			
40			
41			
42			
43			
44			
45			
46			
47			
48			
49			
50			
51			
52			

Total Mileage: _____

Weekly Average for Year: _____

Total Mileage Previous Year: _____

TRAINING MILEAGE GRAPH

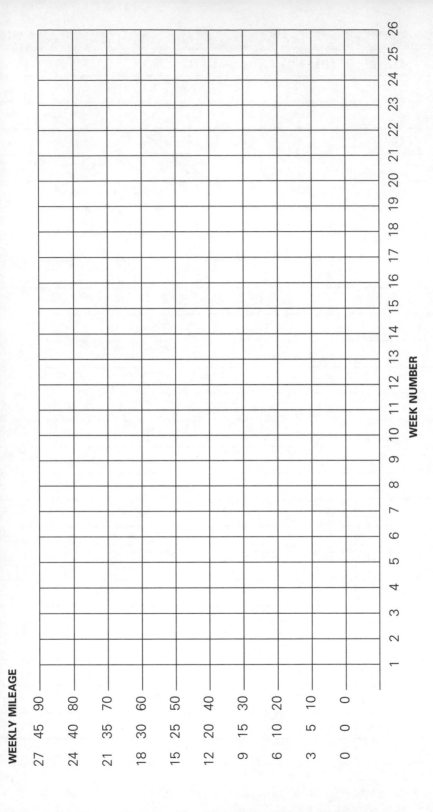

WEEKLY MILEAGE

WEEK NUMBER

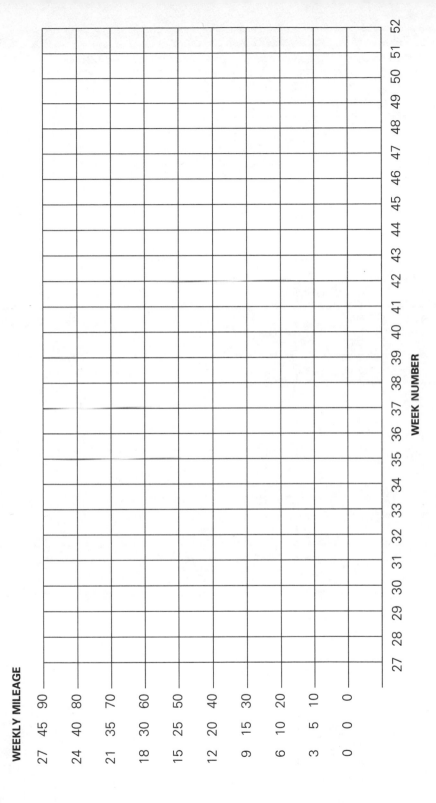

WEEKLY MILEAGE

WEEK NUMBER

KEY LONG-DISTANCE RUNS

DATE	DISTANCE	TIME	PACE	COURSE/COMMENTS

KEY SPEED WORKOUTS

DATE	DIST/REPS	TIMES	AVG. TIME	RECOVERY	COMMENTS

FAVORITE COURSES

COURSE

DATE	TIME	COMMENT

COURSE

DATE	TIME	COMMENT

COURSE

DATE	TIME	COMMENT

COURSE

DATE	TIME	COMMENT

COURSE				COURSE		
DATE	TIME	COMMENT		DATE	TIME	COMMENT

COURSE				COURSE		
DATE	TIME	COMMENT		DATE	TIME	COMMENT

INJURY CHART

INJURY	DATES	CAUSES/TNG CHANGES	TREATMENT	COMMENTS

PART II

Racing

RECORD OF RACES

DATE	RACE	RACE TIMES					1/2 MARA.
		5K	4M	5M	10K	10M	13.1M

MARATHON	MISC	MISC	PACE	RATING	PLACE	COMMENTS/EXCUSES

PERSONAL RECORDS (PRs)

DISTANCE	TIME	RATING	DATE	RACE	COMMENTS
5K					
8K					
10K					
15K					
20K					
MARA.					

DISTANCE	TIME	RATING	DATE	RACE	COMMENTS
MILE					
2 MILES					
4 MILES					
10 MILES					
½ MARA.					
OTHER					

Pacing Chart

PACE PER MILE

How to Use

This chart calculates what pace you race per mile for the most common racing distances—both in miles and kilometers. It can be used these ways:

1. *As a guide to even pacing.* For example, if you wish to run an even pace at 7 minutes per mile for a marathon race, your "splits" should be: 5 miles—35:00; 10 miles—1:10; half marathon—1:31:42; 15 miles—1:45:00; 20 miles—2:20:00; and at the marathon finish—3:03:32.

2. *To help you select a starting pace.* If you wish to break 3½ hours for the marathon, for example, you can refer to the chart and find that this means you must average 8 minutes per mile. Thus you may choose to go out right at 8:00 pace, or perhaps at 7:50 per mile.

3. *To determine your average pace per mile for the race after you have finished.* If you ran 45:21 for 10K, for example, the chart indicates that you averaged 7:18 per mile.

(Times on this chart are in minutes:seconds or hours:minutes:seconds. Example—49:43, 3:29:45.)

PACING CHART

1M	2 M	3 M	4 M	5 M	10 M	1/2 Marathon 13.1 M	15 M	20 M	Marathon 26.22M
0:05:00	0:10:00	0:15:00	0:20:00	0:25:00	0:50:00	1:05:30	1:15:00	1:40:00	2:11:06
0:05:05	0:10:10	0:15:15	0:20:20	0:25:25	0:50:50	1:06:36	1:16:15	1:41:40	2:13:17
0:05:10	0:10:20	0:15:30	0:20:40	0:25:50	0:51:40	1:07:41	1:17:30	1:43:20	2:15:28
0:05:15	0:10:30	0:15:45	0:21:00	0:26:15	0:52:30	1:08:47	1:18:45	1:45:00	2:17:39
0:05:20	0:10:40	0:16:00	0:21:20	0:26:40	0:53:20	1:09:52	1:20:00	1:46:40	2:19:50
0:05:25	0:10:50	0:16:15	0:21:40	0:27:05	0:54:10	1:10:58	1:21:15	1:48:20	2:22:02
0:05:30	0:11:00	0:16:30	0:22:00	0:27:30	0:55:00	1:12:03	1:22:30	1:50:00	2:24:13
0:05:35	0:11:10	0:16:45	0:22:20	0:27:55	0:55:50	1:13:09	1:23:45	1:51:40	2:26:24
0:05:40	1:11:20	0:17:00	0:22:40	0:28:20	0:56:40	1:14:14	1:25:00	1:53:20	2:28:35
0:05:45	0:11:30	0:17:15	0:23:00	0:28:45	0:57:30	1:15:20	1:26:15	1:55:00	2:30:46
0:05:50	0:11:40	0:17:30	0:23:20	0:29:10	0:58:20	1:16:25	1:27:30	1:56:40	2:32:57
0:05:55	0:11:50	0:17:45	0:23:40	0:29:35	0:59:10	1:17:31	1:28:45	1:58:20	2:35:08
0:06:00	0:12:00	0:18:00	0:24:00	0:30:00	1:00:00	1:18:36	1:30:00	2:00:00	2:37:19
0:06:05	0:12:10	0:18:15	0:24:20	0:30:25	1:00:50	1:19:42	1:31:15	2:01:40	2:39:30
0:06:10	0:12:20	0:18:30	0:24:40	0:30:50	1:01:40	1:20:47	1:32:30	2:03:20	2:41:41
0:06:15	0:12:30	0:18:45	0:25:00	0:31:15	1:02:30	1:21:53	1:33:45	2:05:00	2:43:53
0:06:20	0:12:40	0:19:00	0:25:20	0:31:40	1:03:20	1:22:58	1:35:00	2:06:40	2:46:04
0:06:25	0:12:50	0:19:15	0:25:40	0:32:05	1:04:10	1:24:04	1:36:15	2:08:20	2:48:15
0:06:30	0:13:00	0:19:30	0:26:00	0:32:30	1:05:00	1:25:09	1:37:30	2:10:00	2:50:26
0:06:35	0:13:10	0:19:45	0:26:20	0:32:55	1:05:50	1:26:15	1:38:45	2:11:40	2:52:37
0:06:40	0:13:20	0:20:00	0:26:40	0:33:20	1:06:40	1:27:20	1:40:00	2:13:20	2:54:48
0:06:45	0:13:30	0:20:15	0:27:00	0:33:45	1:07:30	1:28:26	1:41:15	2:15:00	2:56:59
0:06:50	0:13:40	0:20:30	0:27:20	0:34:10	1:08:20	1:29:31	1:42:30	2:16:40	2:59:10
0:06:55	0:13:50	0:20:45	0:27:40	0:34:35	1:09:10	1:30:37	1:43:45	2:18:20	3:01:21
0:07:00	0:14:00	0:21:00	0:28:00	0:35:00	1:10:00	1:31:42	1:45:00	2:20:00	3:03:32
0:07:05	0:14:10	0:21:15	0:28:20	0:35:25	1:10:50	1:32:48	1:46:15	2:21:40	3:05:44
0:07:10	0:14:20	0:21:30	0:28:40	0:35:50	1:11:40	1:33:53	1:47:30	2:23:20	3:07:55
0:07:15	0:14:30	0:21:45	0:29:00	0:36:15	1:12:30	1:34:59	1:48:45	2:25:00	3:10:06
0:07:20	0:14:40	0:22:00	0:29:20	0:36:40	1:13:20	1:36:04	1:50:00	2:26:40	3:12:17
0:07:25	0:14:50	0:22:15	0:29:40	0:37:05	1:14:10	1:37:10	1:51:15	2:28:20	3:14:28
0:07:30	0:15:00	0:22:30	0:30:00	0:37:30	1:15:00	1:38:15	1:52:30	2:30:00	3:16:39
0:07:35	0:15:10	0:22:45	0:30:20	0:37:55	1:15:50	1:39:21	1:53:45	2:31:40	3:18:50
0:07:40	0:15:20	0:23:00	0:30:40	0:38:20	1:16:40	1:40:26	1:55:00	2:33:20	3:21:01
0:07:45	0:15:30	0:23:15	0:31:00	0:38:45	1:17:30	1:41:32	1:56:15	2:35:00	3:23:12
0:07:50	0:15:40	0:23:30	0:31:20	0:39:10	1:18:20	1:42:37	1:57:30	2:36:40	3:25:23
0:07:55	0:15:50	0:23:45	0:31:40	0:39:35	1:19:10	1:43:43	1:58:45	2:38:20	3:27:35
0:08:00	0:16:00	0:24:00	0:32:00	0:40:00	1:20:00	1:44:48	2:00:00	2:40:00	3:29:46
0:08:05	0:16:10	0:24:15	0:32:20	0:40:25	1:20:50	1:45:54	2:01:15	2:41:40	3:31:57
0:08:10	0:16:20	0:24:30	0:32:40	0:40:50	1:21:40	1:46:59	2:02:30	2:43:20	3:34:08
0:08:15	0:16:30	0:24:45	0:33:00	0:41:15	1:22:30	1:48:05	2:03:45	2:45:00	3:36:19
0:08:20	0:16:40	0:25:00	0:33:20	0:41:40	1:23:20	1:49:10	2:05:00	2:46:40	3:38:30
0:08:25	0:16:50	0:25:15	0:33:40	0:42:05	1:24:10	1:50:16	2:06:15	2:48:20	3:40:41
0:08:30	0:17:00	0:25:30	0:34:00	0:42:30	1:25:00	1:51:21	2:07:30	2:50:00	3:42:52
0:08:35	0:17:10	0:25:45	0:34:20	0:42:55	1:25:50	1:52:27	2:08:45	2:51:40	3:45:03
0:08:40	0:17:20	0:26:00	0:34:40	0:43:20	1:26:40	1:53:32	2:10:00	2:53:20	3:47:14
0:08:45	0:17:30	0:26:15	0:35:00	0:43:45	1:27:30	1:54:38	2:11:15	2:55:00	3:49:26
0:08:50	0:17:40	0:26:30	0:35:20	0:44:10	1:28:20	1:55:43	2:12:30	2:56:40	3:51:37
0:08:55	0:17:50	0:26:45	0:35:40	0:44:35	1:29:10	1:56:49	2:13:45	2:58:20	3:53:48
0:09:00	0:18:00	0:27:00	0:36:00	0:45:00	1:30:00	1:57:54	2:15:00	3:00:00	3:55:59

1 M	5K	10K	15K	20K	1/2 Marathon 21.1K	25K	30K	Marathon 42.2K
0:05:00	0:15:32	0:31:05	0:46:37	1:02:09	1:05:30	1:18:08	1:33:14	2:11:06
0:05:05	0:15:48	0:31:36	0:47:23	1:03:11	1:06:36	1:19:26	1:34:47	2:13:17
0:05:10	0:16:03	0:32:07	0:48:10	1:04:13	1:07:41	1:20:44	1:36:20	2:15:28
0:05:15	0:16:19	0:32:38	0:48:57	1:05:15	1:08:47	1:22:02	1:37:53	2:17:39
0:05:20	0:16:34	0:33:09	0:49:43	1:06:18	1:09:52	1:23:20	1:39:26	2:19:50
0:05:25	0:16:50	0:33:40	0:50:30	1:07:20	1:10:58	1:24:38	1:41:00	2:22:02
0:05:30	0:17:05	0:34:11	0:51:16	1:08:22	1:12:03	1:25:56	1:42:33	2:24:13
0:05:35	0:17:21	0:34:42	0:52:03	1:09:24	1:13:09	1:27:14	1:44:06	2:26:24
0:05:40	0:17:37	0:35:13	0:52:50	1:10:26	1:14:14	1:28:33	1:45:39	2:28:35
0:05:45	0:17:52	0:35:44	0:53:36	1:11:28	1:15:20	1:29:51	1:47:13	2:30:46
0:05:50	0:18:08	0:36:15	0:54:23	1:12:31	1:16:25	1:31:09	1:48:46	2:32:57
0:05:55	0:18:23	0:36:46	0:55:10	1:13:33	1:17:31	1:32:27	1:50:19	2:35:08
0:06:00	0:18:39	0:37:17	0:55:56	1:14:35	1:18:36	1:33:45	1:51:52	2:37:19
0:06:05	0:18:54	0:37:48	0:56:43	1:15:37	1:19:42	1:35:03	1:53:25	2:39:30
0:06:10	0:19:10	0:38:20	0:57:29	1:16:39	1:20:47	1:36:21	1:54:59	2:41:41
0:06:15	0:19:25	0:38:51	0:58:16	1:17:41	1:21:53	1:37:39	1:56:32	2:43:53
0:06:20	0:19:41	0:39:22	0:59:03	1:18:43	1:22:58	1:38:58	1:58:05	2:46:04
0:06:25	0:19:56	0:39:53	0:59:49	1:19:46	1:24:04	1:40:16	1:59:38	2:48:15
0:06:30	0:20:12	0:40:24	1:00:36	1:20:48	1:25:09	1:41:34	2:01:12	2:50:26
0:06:35	0:20:27	0:40:55	1:01:22	1:21:50	1:26:15	1:42:52	2:02:45	2:52:37
0:06:40	0:20:43	0:41:26	1:02:09	1:22:52	1:27:20	1:44:10	2:04:18	2:54:48
0:06:45	0:20:59	0:41:57	1:02:56	1:23:54	1:28:26	1:45:28	2:05:51	2:56:59
0:06:50	0:21:14	0:42:28	1:03:42	1:24:56	1:29:31	1:46:46	2:07:24	2:59:10
0:06:55	0:21:30	0:42:59	1:04:29	1:25:58	1:30:37	1:48:04	2:08:58	3:01:21
0:07:00	0:21:45	0:43:30	1:05:15	1:27:01	1:31:42	1:49:23	2:10:31	3:03:32
0:07:05	0:22:01	0:44:01	1:06:02	1:28:03	1:32:48	1:50:41	2:12:04	3:05:44
0:07:10	0:22:16	0:44:32	1:06:49	1:29:05	1:33:53	1:51:59	2:13:37	3:07:55
0:07:15	0:22:32	0:45:04	1:07:35	1:30:07	1:34:59	1:53:17	2:15:11	3:10:06
0:07:20	0:22:47	0:45:35	1:08:22	1:31:09	1:36:04	1:54:35	2:16:44	3:12:17
0:07:25	0:23:03	0:46:06	1:09:09	1:32:11	1:37:10	1:55:53	2:18:17	3:14:28
0:07:30	0:23:18	0:46:37	1:09:55	1:33:14	1:38:15	1:57:11	2:19:50	3:16:39
0:07:35	0:23:34	0:47:08	1:10:42	1:34:16	1:39:21	1:58:29	2:21:24	3:18:50
0:07:40	0:23:49	0:47:39	1:11:28	1:35:18	1:40:26	1:59:48	2:22:57	3:21:01
0:07:45	0:24:05	0:48:10	1:12:15	1:36:20	1:41:32	2:01:06	2:24:30	3:23:12
0:07:50	0:24:21	0:48:41	1:13:02	1:37:22	1:42:37	2:02:24	2:26:03	3:25:23
0:07:55	0:24:36	0:49:12	1:13:48	1:38:24	1:43:43	2:03:42	2:27:36	3:27:35
0:08:00	0:24:52	0:49:43	1:14:35	1:39:26	1:44:48	2:05:00	2:29:10	3:29:46
0:08:05	0:25:07	0:50:14	1:15:21	1:40:29	1:45:54	2:06:18	2:30:43	3:31:57
0:08:10	0:25:23	0:50:45	1:16:08	1:41:31	1:46:59	2:07:36	2:32:16	3:34:08
0:08:15	0:25:38	0:51:16	1:16:55	1:42:33	1:48:05	2:08:54	2:33:49	3:36:19
0:08:20	0:25:54	0:51:48	1:17:41	1:43:35	1:49:10	2:10:13	2:35:23	3:38:30
0:08:25	0:26:09	0:52:19	1:18:28	1:44:37	1:50:16	2:11:31	2:36:56	3:40:41
0:08:30	0:26:25	0:52:50	1:19:15	1:45:39	1:51:21	2:12:49	2:38:29	3:42:52
0:08:35	0:26:40	0:53:21	1:20:01	1:46:41	1:52:27	2:14:07	2:40:02	3:45:03
0:08:40	0:26:56	0:53:52	1:20:48	1:47:44	1:53:32	2:15:25	2:41:35	3:47:14
0:08:45	0:27:11	0:54:23	1:21:34	1:48:46	1:54:38	2:16:43	2:43:09	3:49:26
0:08:50	0:27:27	0:54:54	1:22:21	1:49:48	1:55:43	2:18:01	2:44:42	3:51:37
0:08:55	0:27:43	0:55:25	1:23:08	1:50:50	1:56:49	2:19:19	2:46:15	3:53:48
0:09:00	0:27:58	0:55:56	1:23:54	1:51:52	1:57:54	2:20:38	2:47:48	3:55:59

1M	2 M	3 M	4 M	5 M	10 M	1/2 Marathon 13.1 M	15 M	20 M	Marathon 26.22M
0:09:05	0:18:10	0:27:15	0:36:20	0:45:25	1:30:50	1:59:00	2:16:15	3:01:40	3:58:10
0:09:10	0:18:20	0:27:30	0:36:40	0:45:50	1:31:40	2:00:05	2:17:30	3:03:20	4:00:21
0:09:15	0:18:30	0:27:45	0:37:00	0:46:15	1:32:30	2:01:11	2:18:45	3:05:00	4:02:32
0:09:20	0:18:40	0:28:00	0:37:20	0:46:40	1:33:20	2:02:16	2:20:00	3:06:40	4:04:43
0:09:25	0:18:50	0:28:15	0:37:40	0:47:05	1:34:10	2:03:22	2:21:15	3:08:20	4:06:54
0:09:30	0:19:00	0:28:30	0:38:00	0:47:30	1:35:00	2:04:27	2:22:30	3:10:00	4:09:05
0:09:35	0:19:10	0:28:45	0:38:20	0:47:55	1:35:50	2:05:33	2:23:45	3:11:40	4:11:17
0:09:40	0:19:20	0:29:00	0:38:40	0:48:20	1:36:40	2:06:38	2:25:00	3:13:20	4:13:28
0:09:45	0:19:30	0:29:15	0:39:00	0:48:45	1:37:30	2:07:44	2:26:15	3:15:00	4:15:39
0:09:50	0:19:40	0:29:30	0:39:20	0:49:10	1:38:20	2:08:49	2:27:30	3:16:40	4:17:50
0:09:55	0:19:50	0:29:45	0:39:40	0:49:35	1:39:10	2:09:55	2:28:45	3:18:20	4:20:01
0:10:00	0:20:00	0:30:00	0:40:00	0:50:00	1:40:00	2:11:00	2:30:00	3:20:00	4:22:12
0:10:05	0:20:10	0:30:15	0:40:20	0:50:25	1:40:50	2:12:06	2:31:15	3:21:40	4:24:23
0:10:10	0:20:20	0:30:30	0:40:40	0:50:50	1:41:40	2:13:11	2:32:30	3:23:20	4:26:34
0:10:15	0:20:30	0:30:45	0:41:00	0:51:15	1:42:30	2:14:17	2:33:45	3:25:00	4:28:45
0:10:20	0:20:40	0:31:00	0:41:20	0:51:40	1:43:20	2:15:22	2:35:00	3:26:40	4:30:56
0:10:25	0:20:50	0:31:15	0:41:40	0:52:05	1:44:10	2:16:28	2:36:15	3:28:20	4:33:08
0:10:30	0:21:00	0:31:30	0:42:00	0:52:30	1:45:00	2:17:33	2:37:30	3:30:00	4:35:19
0:10:35	0:21:10	0:31:45	0:42:20	0:52:55	1:45:50	2:18:39	2:38:45	3:31:40	4:37:30
0:10:40	0:21:20	0:32:00	0:42:40	0:53:20	1:46:40	2:19:44	2:40:00	3:33:20	4:39:41
0:10:45	0:21:30	0:32:15	0:43:00	0:53:45	1:47:30	2:20:50	2:41:15	3:35:00	4:41:52
0:10:50	0:21:40	0:32:30	0:43:20	0:54:10	1:48:20	2:21:55	2:42:30	3:36:40	4:44:03
0:10:55	0:21:50	0:32:45	0:43:40	0:54:35	1:49:10	2:23:01	2:43:45	3:38:20	4:46:14
0:11:00	0:22:00	0:33:00	0:44:00	0:55:00	1:50:00	2:24:06	2:45:00	3:40:00	4:48:25
0:11:05	0:22:10	0:33:15	0:44:20	0:55:25	1:50:50	2:25:12	2:46:15	3:41:40	4:50:36
0:11:10	0:22:20	0:33:30	0:44:40	0:55:50	1:51:40	2:26:17	2:47:30	3:43:20	4:52:47
0:11:15	0:22:30	0:33:45	0:45:00	0:56:15	1:52:30	2:27:23	2:48:45	3:45:00	4:54:59
0:11:20	0:22:40	0:34:00	0:45:20	0:56:40	1:53:20	2:28:28	2:50:00	3:46:40	4:57:10
0:11:25	0:22:50	0:34:15	0:45:40	0:57:05	1:54:10	2:29:34	2:51:15	3:48:20	4:59:21
0:11:30	0:23:00	0:34:30	0:46:00	0:57:30	1:55:00	2:30:39	2:52:30	3:50:00	5:01:32
0:11:35	0:23:10	0:34:45	0:46:20	0:57:55	1:55:50	2:31:45	2:53:45	3:51:40	5:03:43
0:11:40	0:23:20	0:35:00	0:46:40	0:58:20	1:56:40	2:32:50	2:55:00	3:53:20	5:05:54
0:11:45	0:23:30	0:35:15	0:47:00	0:58:45	1:57:30	2:33:56	2:56:15	3:55:00	5:08:05
0:11:50	0:23:40	0:35:30	0:47:20	0:59:10	1:58:20	2:35:01	2:57:30	3:56:40	5:10:16
0:11:55	0:23:50	0:35:45	0:47:40	0:59:35	1:59:10	2:36:07	2:58:45	3:58:20	5:12:27
0:12:00	0:24:00	0:36:00	0:48:00	1:00:00	2:00:00	2:37:12	3:00:00	4:00:00	5:14:38
0:12:05	0:24:10	0:36:15	0:48:20	1:00:25	2:00:50	2:38:18	3:01:15	4:01:40	5:16:50
0:12:10	0:24:20	0:36:30	0:48:40	1:00:50	2:01:40	2:39:23	3:02:30	4:03:20	5:19:01
0:12:15	0:24:30	0:36:45	0:49:00	1:01:15	2:02:30	2:40:29	3:03:45	4:05:00	5:21:12
0:12:20	0:24:40	0:37:00	0:49:20	1:01:40	2:03:20	2:41:34	3:05:00	4:06:40	5:23:23
0:12:25	0:24:50	0:37:15	0:49:40	1:02:05	2:04:10	2:42:40	3:06:15	4:08:20	5:25:34
0:12:30	0:25:00	0:37:30	0:50:00	1:02:30	2:05:00	2:43:45	3:07:30	4:10:00	5:27:45
0:12:35	0:25:10	0:37:45	0:50:20	1:02:55	2:05:50	2:44:51	3:08:45	4:11:40	5:29:56
0:12:40	0:25:20	0:38:00	0:50:40	1:03:20	2:06:40	2:45:56	3:10:00	4:13:20	5:32:07
0:12:45	0:25:30	0:38:15	0:51:00	1:03:45	2:07:30	2:47:02	3:11:15	4:15:00	5:34:18
0:12:50	0:25:40	0:38:30	0:51:20	1:04:10	2:08:20	2:48:07	3:12:30	4:16:40	5:36:29
0:12:55	0:25:50	0:38:45	0:51:40	1:04:35	2:09:10	2:49:13	3:13:45	4:18:20	5:38:40
0:13:00	0:26:00	0:39:00	0:52:00	1:05:00	2:10:00	2:50:18	3:15:00	4:20:00	5:40:52

1 M	5K	10K	15K	20K	1/2 Marathon 21.1K	25K	30K	Marathon 42.2K
0:09:05	0:28:14	0:56:27	1:24:41	1:52:54	1:59:00	2:21:56	2:49:22	3:58:10
0:09:10	0:28:29	0:56:58	1:25:27	1:53:57	2:00:05	2:23:14	2:50:55	4:00:21
0:09:15	0:28:45	0:57:29	1:26:14	1:54:59	2:01:11	2:24:32	2:52:28	4:02:32
0:09:20	0:29:00	0:58:00	1:27:01	1:56:01	2:02:16	2:25:50	2:54:01	4:04:43
0:09:25	0:29:16	0:58:31	1:27:47	1:57:03	2:03:22	2:27:08	2:55:34	4:06:54
0:09:30	0:29:31	0:59:03	1:28:34	1:58:05	2:04:27	2:28:26	2:57:08	4:09:05
0:09:35	0:29:47	0:59:34	1:29:20	1:59:07	2:05:33	2:29:44	2:58:41	4:11:17
0:09:40	0:30:02	1:00:05	1:30:07	2:00:09	2:06:38	2:31:03	3:00:14	4:13:28
0:09:45	0:30:18	1:00:36	1:30:54	2:01:12	2:07:44	2:32:21	3:01:47	4:15:39
0:09:50	0:30:33	1:01:07	1:31:40	2:02:14	2:08:49	2:33:39	3:03:21	4:17:50
0:09:55	0:30:49	1:01:38	1:32:27	2:03:16	2:09:55	2:34:57	3:04:54	4:20:01
0:10:00	0:31:05	1:02:09	1:33:14	2:04:18	2:11:00	2:36:15	3:06:27	4:22:12
0:10:05	0:31:20	1:02:40	1:34:00	2:05:20	2:12:06	2:37:33	3:08:00	4:24:23
0:10:10	0:31:36	1:03:11	1:34:47	2:06:22	2:13:11	2:38:51	3:09:34	4:26:34
0:10:15	0:31:51	1:03:42	1:35:33	2:07:24	2:14:17	2:40:09	3:11:07	4:28:45
0:10:20	0:32:07	1:04:13	1:36:20	2:08:27	2:15:22	2:41:28	3:12:40	4:30:56
0:10:25	0:32:22	1:04:44	1:37:07	2:09:29	2:16:28	2:42:46	3:14:13	4:33:08
0:10:30	0:32:38	1:05:15	1:37:53	2:10:31	2:17:33	2:44:04	3:15:46	4:35:19
0:10:35	0:32:53	1:05:47	1:38:40	2:11:33	2:18:39	2:45:22	3:17:20	4:37:30
0:10:40	0:33:09	1:06:18	1:39:26	2:12:35	2:19:44	2:46:40	3:18:53	4:39:41
0:10:45	0:33:24	1:06:49	1:40:13	2:13:37	2:20:50	2:47:58	3:20:26	4:41:52
0:10:50	0:33:40	1:07:20	1:41:00	2:14:40	2:21:55	2:49:16	3:21:59	4:44:03
0:10:55	0:33:55	1:07:51	1:41:46	2:15:42	2:23:01	2:50:34	3:23:33	4:46:14
0:11:00	0:34:11	1:08:22	1:42:33	2:16:44	2:24:06	2:51:53	3:25:06	4:48:25
0:11:05	0:34:27	1:08:53	1:43:20	2:17:46	2:25:12	2:53:11	3:26:39	4:50:36
0:11:10	0:34:42	1:09:24	1:44:06	2:18:48	2:26:17	2:54:29	3:28:12	4:52:47
0:11:15	0:34:58	1:09:55	1:44:53	2:19:50	2:27:23	2:55:47	3:29:45	4:54:59
0:11:20	0:35:13	1:10:26	1:45:39	2:20:52	2:28:28	2:57:05	3:31:19	4:57:10
0:11:25	0:35:29	1:10:57	1:46:26	2:21:55	2:29:34	2:58:23	3:32:52	4:59:21
0:11:30	0:35:44	1:11:28	1:47:13	2:22:57	2:30:39	2:59:41	3:34:25	5:01:32
0:11:35	0:36:00	1:11:59	1:47:59	2:23:59	2:31:45	3:00:59	3:35:58	5:03:43
0:11:40	0:36:15	1:12:31	1:48:46	2:25:01	2:32:50	3:02:18	3:37:32	5:05:54
0:11:45	0:36:31	1:13:02	1:49:32	2:26:03	2:33:56	3:03:36	3:39:05	5:08:05
0:11:50	0:36:46	1:13:33	1:50:19	2:27:05	2:35:01	3:04:54	3:40:38	5:10:16
0:11:55	0:37:02	1:14:04	1:51:06	2:28:08	2:36:07	3:06:12	3:42:11	5:12:27
0:12:00	0:37:17	1:14:35	1:51:52	2:29:10	2:37:12	3:07:30	3:43:44	5:14:38
0:12:05	0:37:33	1:15:06	1:52:39	2:30:12	2:38:18	3:08:48	3:45:18	5:16:50
0:12:10	0:37:48	1:15:37	1:53:25	2:31:14	2:39:23	3:10:06	3:46:51	5:19:01
0:12:15	0:38:04	1:16:08	1:54:12	2:32:16	2:40:29	3:11:24	3:48:24	5:21:12
0:12:20	0:38:20	1:16:39	1:54:59	2:33:18	2:41:34	3:12:43	3:49:57	5:23:23
0:12:25	0:38:35	1:17:10	1:55:45	2:34:20	2:42:40	3:14:01	3:51:31	5:25:34
0:12:30	0:38:51	1:17:41	1:56:32	2:35:23	2:43:45	3:15:19	3:53:04	5:27:45
0:12:35	0:39:06	1:18:12	1:57:19	2:36:25	2:44:51	3:16:37	3:54:37	5:29:56
0:12:40	0:39:22	1:18:43	1:58:05	2:37:27	2:45:56	3:17:55	3:56:10	5:32:07
0:12:45	0:39:37	1:19:15	1:58:52	2:38:29	2:47:02	3:19:13	3:57:44	5:34:18
0:12:50	0:39:53	1:19:46	1:59:38	2:39:31	2:48:07	3:20:31	3:59:17	5:36:29
0:12:55	0:40:08	1:20:17	2:00:25	2:40:33	2:49:13	3:21:49	4:00:50	5:38:40
0:13:00	0:40:24	1:20:48	2:01:12	2:41:35	2:50:18	3:23:08	4:02:23	5:40:52

Race Time Comparison and Predictor Charts

These performance charts establish scores for runners of all ages and ability levels at popular race distances from 5K to the marathon. A perfect score is 1,000 points, which is 100 percent of the world record for each race distance when the charts were compiled. All other scores represent a percentage of this standard. For example, 510 points for a male runner who runs 25:25 for 5K is 51 percent of the world record standard time of 12:58.4.

The charts can be used for two important purposes:

1. **Rate your best performances for all distances.** You can compare your scores between different race distances to determine your best racing distance or range (such as 5K–10K, or ½ marathon–marathon). Use the chart to compare lifetime personal records as well as best times for each racing season. The charts may reveal more ability or better training at certain distances. Example: A male runner scores 600 points for 5K, 570 points for 10K, and 520 points for the marathon. He obviously is faster and, most likely, better trained for the shorter distance. Record your performance score for each race under the rating column for the Record of Races chart on page 126 and the Personal Records chart on page 128.

2. **Predict race times and establish race goals.** If your training is of equal quality for different distances, you can predict your race time from a recent race. For example, a woman runs 21:03 for

a 5K a month prior to a 10K race. That is a 720-point-value performance equal to a 41:17 for 10K. Thus she can use this information to establish her race time goal and starting pace.

The predictor charts are more accurate the closer the racing distances. For example, it is much more accurate to predict a 5-mile or 10K result from a 5K race than from a marathon, or a marathon from a ½ marathon than from a mile.

When making time comparisons, you should adjust for weather conditions (heat, humidity, cold, altitude, wind) as well as course conditions (hills, surface, turns, footing). These charts are based purely on race time statistics and should be used as a general guide. Masters runners may use the following age-adjusted charts to compare and predict race times.

NOTE: If your race time falls between two point scores, either round off to the nearest score or interpolate to establish an intermediate score. For example, a male running 21:00 for 5K is nearest to the 620 score; or he can interpolate and give himself a score of 618.

MEN'S RACE TIME COMPARISON AND PREDICTOR CHART

RATING	5K	8K/5M	10K	15K	10M	20K	1/2 Marathon	Marathon
1000	0:12:58	0:21:19	0:26:58	0:41:26	0:44:40	0:56:20	0:59:03	2:06:50
990	0:13:06	0:21:32	0:27:14	0:41:51	0:45:07	0:56:54	0:59:39	2:08:07
980	0:13:14	0:21:45	0:27:31	0:42:17	0:45:35	0:57:29	1:00:15	2:09:25
970	0:13:22	0:21:59	0:27:48	0:42:43	0:46:03	0:58:05	1:00:53	2:10:45
960	0:13:30	0:22:12	0:28:05	0:43:10	0:46:32	0:58:41	1:01:31	2:12:07
950	0:13:39	0:22:26	0:28:23	0:43:37	0:47:01	0:59:18	1:02:09	2:13:31
940	0:13:48	0:22:41	0:28:41	0:44:05	0:47:31	0:59:56	1:02:49	2:14:56
930	0:13:57	0:22:55	0:29:00	0:44:33	0:48:02	1:00:34	1:03:30	2:16:23
920	0:14:06	0:23:10	0:29:19	0:45:02	0:48:33	1:01:14	1:04:11	2:17:52
910	0:14:15	0:23:25	0:29:38	0:45:32	0:49:05	1:01:54	1:04:53	2:19:23
900	0:14:24	0:23:41	0:29:58	0:46:02	0:49:38	1:02:36	1:05:37	2:20:56
890	0:14:34	0:23:57	0:30:18	0:46:33	0:50:11	1:03:18	1:06:21	2:22:31
880	0:14:44	0:24:13	0:30:39	0:47:05	0:50:45	1:04:01	1:07:06	2:24:08
870	0:14:54	0:24:30	0:31:00	0:47:37	0:51:20	1:04:45	1:07:52	2:25:47
860	0:15:05	0:24:47	0:31:21	0:48:11	0:51:56	1:05:30	1:08:40	2:27:29
850	0:15:15	0:25:05	0:31:44	0:48:45	0:52:33	1:06:16	1:09:28	2:29:13
840	0:15:26	0:25:23	0:32:06	0:49:20	0:53:10	1:07:04	1:10:18	2:31:00
830	0:15:37	0:25:41	0:32:29	0:49:55	0:53:49	1:07:52	1:11:09	2:32:49
820	0:15:49	0:26:00	0:32:53	0:50:32	0:54:28	1:08:42	1:12:01	2:34:40
810	0:16:00	0:26:19	0:33:18	0:51:09	0:55:09	1:09:33	1:12:54	2:36:35
800	0:16:12	0:26:39	0:33:42	0:51:47	0:55:50	1:10:25	1:13:49	2:38:32
795	0:16:19	0:26:49	0:33:55	0:52:07	0:56:11	1:10:52	1:14:17	2:39:32
790	0:16:25	0:26:59	0:34:08	0:52:27	0:56:32	1:11:18	1:14:45	2:40:33
785	0:16:31	0:27:09	0:34:21	0:52:47	0:56:54	1:11:46	1:15:13	2:41:34
780	0:16:37	0:27:20	0:34:34	0:53:07	0:57:16	1:12:13	1:15:42	2:42:36
775	0:16:44	0:27:30	0:34:48	0:53:28	0:57:38	1:12:41	1:16:12	2:43:39
770	0:16:50	0:27:41	0:35:01	0:53:49	0:58:01	1:13:10	1:16:41	2:44:43
765	0:16:57	0:27:52	0:35:15	0:54:10	0:58:23	1:13:38	1:17:11	2:45:48
760	0:17:04	0:28:03	0:35:29	0:54:31	0:58:46	1:14:07	1:17:42	2:46:53
755	0:17:10	0:28:14	0:35:43	0:54:53	0:59:10	1:14:37	1:18:13	2:47:59
750	0:17:17	0:28:25	0:35:57	0:55:15	0:59:33	1:15:07	1:18:44	2:49:07
745	0:17:24	0:28:37	0:36:12	0:55:37	0:59:57	1:15:37	1:19:16	2:50:15
740	0:17:31	0:28:48	0:36:26	0:55:59	1:00:22	1:16:08	1:19:48	2:51:24
735	0:17:39	0:29:00	0:36:41	0:56:22	1:00:46	1:16:39	1:20:20	2:52:34
730	0:17:46	0:29:12	0:36:56	0:56:45	1:01:11	1:17:10	1:20:53	2:53:45
725	0:17:53	0:29:24	0:37:12	0:57:09	1:01:37	1:17:42	1:21:27	2:54:57
720	0:18:01	0:29:36	0:37:27	0:57:33	1:02:02	1:18:14	1:22:01	2:56:09
715	0:18:08	0:29:49	0:37:43	0:57:57	1:02:28	1:18:47	1:22:35	2:57:23
710	0:18:16	0:30:01	0:37:59	0:58:21	1:02:55	1:19:21	1:23:10	2:58:38
705	0:18:24	0:30:14	0:38:15	0:58:46	1:03:21	1:19:54	1:23:46	2:59:54
700	0:18:31	0:30:27	0:38:31	0:59:11	1:03:49	1:20:29	1:24:21	3:01:11
695	0:18:39	0:30:40	0:38:48	0:59:37	1:04:16	1:21:03	1:24:58	3:02:30
690	0:18:48	0:30:54	0:39:05	1:00:03	1:04:44	1:21:39	1:25:35	3:03:49
685	0:18:56	0:31:07	0:39:22	1:00:29	1:05:12	1:22:14	1:26:12	3:05:09
680	0:19:04	0:31:21	0:39:39	1:00:56	1:05:41	1:22:51	1:26:50	3:06:31
675	0:19:13	0:31:35	0:39:57	1:01:23	1:06:10	1:23:27	1:27:29	3:07:54
670	0:19:21	0:31:49	0:40:15	1:01:50	1:06:40	1:24:05	1:28:08	3:09:18
665	0:19:30	0:32:03	0:40:33	1:02:18	1:07:10	1:24:43	1:28:48	3:10:44
660	0:19:39	0:32:18	0:40:52	1:02:47	1:07:41	1:25:21	1:29:28	3:12:10
655	0:19:48	0:32:33	0:41:10	1:03:15	1:08:12	1:26:00	1:30:09	3:13:38
650	0:19:57	0:32:48	0:41:29	1:03:45	1:08:43	1:26:40	1:30:51	3:15:08
645	0:20:06	0:33:03	0:41:49	1:04:14	1:09:15	1:27:20	1:31:33	3:16:38
640	0:20:16	0:33:18	0:42:08	1:04:44	1:09:48	1:28:01	1:32:16	3:18:11

138

RATING	5K	8K/5M	10K	15K	10M	20K	1/2 Marathon	Marathon
635	0:20:25	0:33:34	0:42:28	1:05:15	1:10:20	1:28:43	1:33:00	3:19:44
630	0:20:35	0:33:50	0:42:48	1:05:46	1:10:54	1:29:25	1:33:44	3:21:19
625	0:20:45	0:34:06	0:43:09	1:06:18	1:11:28	1:30:08	1:34:29	3:22:56
620	0:20:55	0:34:23	0:43:30	1:06:50	1:12:03	1:30:52	1:35:15	3:24:34
615	0:21:05	0:34:40	0:43:51	1:07:22	1:12:38	1:31:36	1:36:01	3:26:14
610	0:21:15	0:34:57	0:44:12	1:07:55	1:13:13	1:32:21	1:36:48	3:27:55
605	0:21:26	0:35:14	0:44:34	1:08:29	1:13:50	1:33:07	1:37:36	3:29:39
600	0:21:37	0:35:32	0:44:57	1:09:03	1:14:27	1:33:53	1:38:25	3:31:23
595	0:21:48	0:35:50	0:45:19	1:09:38	1:15:04	1:34:41	1:39:15	3:33:10
590	0:21:59	0:36:08	0:45:42	1:10:14	1:15:42	1:35:29	1:40:05	3:34:58
585	0:22:10	0:36:26	0:46:06	1:10:50	1:16:21	1:36:18	1:40:56	3:36:49
580	0:22:21	0:36:45	0:46:30	1:11:26	1:17:01	1:37:08	1:41:49	3:38:41
575	0:22:33	0:37:04	0:46:54	1:12:03	1:17:41	1:37:58	1:42:42	3:40:35
570	0:22:45	0:37:24	0:47:19	1:12:41	1:18:22	1:38:50	1:43:36	3:42:31
565	0:22:57	0:37:44	0:47:44	1:13:20	1:19:03	1:39:42	1:44:31	3:44:29
560	0:23:09	0:38:04	0:48:09	1:13:59	1:19:46	1:40:36	1:45:27	3:46:29
555	0:23:22	0:38:25	0:48:35	1:14:39	1:20:29	1:41:30	1:46:24	3:48:32
550	0:23:35	0:38:45	0:49:02	1:15:20	1:21:13	1:42:25	1:47:22	3:50:36
545	0:23:48	0:39:07	0:49:29	1:16:01	1:21:57	1:43:22	1:48:21	3:52:43
540	0:24:01	0:39:29	0:49:56	1:16:44	1:22:43	1:44:19	1:49:21	3:54:53
535	0:24:14	0:39:51	0:50:24	1:17:27	1:23:29	1:45:18	1:50:22	3:57:04
530	0:24:28	0:40:13	0:50:53	1:18:11	1:24:17	1:46:17	1:51:25	3:59:18
525	0:24:42	0:40:36	0:51:22	1:18:55	1:25:05	1:47:18	1:52:29	4:01:35
520	0:24:56	0:41:00	0:51:52	1:19:41	1:25:54	1:48:20	1:53:33	4:03:55
515	0:25:11	0:41:23	0:52:22	1:20:27	1:26:44	1:49:23	1:54:40	4:06:17
510	0:25:25	0:41:48	0:52:53	1:21:15	1:27:35	1:50:27	1:55:47	4:08:42
505	0:25:41	0:42:13	0:53:24	1:22:03	1:28:27	1:51:33	1:56:56	4:11:09
500	0:25:56	0:42:38	0:53:56	1:22:52	1:29:20	1:52:40	1:58:06	4:13:40
495	0:26:12	0:43:04	0:54:29	1:23:42	1:30:14	1:53:48	1:59:18	4:16:14
490	0:26:28	0:43:30	0:55:02	1:24:33	1:31:09	1:54:58	2:00:31	4:18:51
485	0:26:44	0:43:57	0:55:36	1:25:26	1:32:06	1:56:09	2:01:45	4:21:31
480	0:27:01	0:44:25	0:56:11	1:26:19	1:33:03	1:57:22	2:03:01	4:24:14
475	0:27:18	0:44:53	0:56:46	1:27:14	1:34:02	1:58:36	2:04:19	4:27:01
470	0:27:35	0:45:21	0:57:23	1:28:09	1:35:02	1:59:51	2:05:38	4:29:51
465	0:27:53	0:45:51	0:58:00	1:29:06	1:36:03	2:01:09	2:06:59	4:32:46
460	0:28:11	0:46:20	0:58:37	1:30:04	1:37:06	2:02:28	2:08:22	4:35:43
455	0:28:30	0:46:51	0:59:16	1:31:04	1:38:10	2:03:49	2:09:47	4:38:45
450	0:28:49	0:47:22	0:59:56	1:32:04	1:39:16	2:05:11	2:11:13	4:41:51
445	0:29:08	0:47:54	1:00:36	1:33:07	1:40:22	2:06:36	2:12:42	4:45:01
440	0:29:28	0:48:27	1:01:17	1:34:10	1:41:31	2:08:02	2:14:12	4:48:15
435	0:29:49	0:49:00	1:02:00	1:35:15	1:42:41	2:09:30	2:15:45	4:51:34
430	0:30:09	0:49:34	1:02:43	1:36:21	1:43:53	2:11:00	2:17:20	4:54:58
425	0:30:31	0:50:09	1:03:27	1:37:29	1:45:06	2:12:33	2:18:56	4:58:26
420	0:30:52	0:50:45	1:04:12	1:38:39	1:46:21	2:14:08	2:20:36	5:01:59
415	0:31:15	0:51:22	1:04:59	1:39:50	1:47:38	2:15:45	2:22:17	5:05:37
410	0:31:38	0:52:00	1:05:46	1:41:03	1:48:57	2:17:24	2:24:01	5:09:21
405	0:32:01	0:52:38	1:06:35	1:42:18	1:50:17	2:19:06	2:25:48	5:13:10
400	0:32:25	0:53:18	1:07:25	1:43:35	1:51:40	2:20:50	2:27:38	5:17:05
395	0:32:50	0:53:58	1:08:16	1:44:54	1:53:05	2:22:37	2:29:30	5:21:06
390	0:33:15	0:54:39	1:09:09	1:46:14	1:54:32	2:24:27	2:31:25	5:25:13
385	0:33:41	0:55:22	1:10:03	1:47:37	1:56:01	2:26:19	2:33:23	5:29:26
380	0:34:07	0:56:06	1:10:58	1:49:02	1:57:33	2:28:15	2:35:24	5:33:46
375	0:34:35	0:56:51	1:11:55	1:50:29	1:59:07	2:30:13	2:37:28	5:38:13

WOMEN'S RACE TIME COMPARISON AND PREDICTOR CHART

RATING	5K	8K/5M	10K	15K	10M	20K	1/2 Marathon	Marathon
1000	0:14:23	0:23:39	0:29:55	0:45:51	0:49:23	1:02:10	1:05:48	2:18:51
990	0:14:32	0:23:53	0:30:13	0:46:19	0:49:53	1:02:48	1:06:28	2:20:15
980	0:14:41	0:24:08	0:30:32	0:46:47	0:50:23	1:03:26	1:07:09	2:21:41
970	0:14:50	0:24:23	0:30:51	0:47:16	0:50:55	1:04:05	1:07:50	2:23:09
960	0:14:59	0:24:38	0:31:10	0:47:46	0:51:26	1:04:45	1:08:32	2:24:38
950	0:15:08	0:24:54	0:31:29	0:48:16	0:51:59	1:05:26	1:09:16	2:26:09
940	0:15:18	0:25:10	0:31:50	0:48:47	0:52:32	1:06:08	1:10:00	2:27:43
930	0:15:28	0:25:26	0:32:10	0:49:18	0:53:06	1:06:51	1:10:45	2:29:18
920	0:15:38	0:25:42	0:32:31	0:49:50	0:53:41	1:07:34	1:11:31	2:30:55
910	0:15:48	0:25:59	0:32:53	0:50:23	0:54:16	1:08:19	1:12:18	2:32:35
900	0:15:59	0:26:17	0:33:14	0:50:57	0:54:52	1:09:04	1:13:07	2:34:17
890	0:16:10	0:26:34	0:33:37	0:51:31	0:55:29	1:09:51	1:13:56	2:36:01
880	0:16:21	0:26:52	0:34:00	0:52:06	0:56:07	1:10:39	1:14:46	2:37:47
870	0:16:32	0:27:11	0:34:23	0:52:42	0:56:46	1:11:27	1:15:38	2:39:36
860	0:16:43	0:27:30	0:34:47	0:53:19	0:57:25	1:12:17	1:16:31	2:41:27
850	0:16:55	0:27:49	0:35:12	0:53:56	0:58:06	1:13:08	1:17:25	2:43:21
840	0:17:07	0:28:09	0:35:37	0:54:35	0:58:47	1:14:00	1:18:20	2:45:18
830	0:17:20	0:28:30	0:36:03	0:55:14	0:59:30	1:14:54	1:19:17	2:47:17
820	0:17:32	0:28:50	0:36:29	0:55:55	1:00:13	1:15:49	1:20:15	2:49:20
810	0:17:45	0:29:12	0:36:56	0:56:36	1:00:58	1:16:45	1:21:14	2:51:25
800	0:17:59	0:29:34	0:37:24	0:57:19	1:01:44	1:17:42	1:22:15	2:53:34
795	0:18:06	0:29:45	0:37:38	0:57:40	1:02:07	1:18:12	1:22:46	2:54:39
790	0:18:12	0:29:56	0:37:52	0:58:02	1:02:31	1:18:42	1:23:17	2:55:46
785	0:18:19	0:30:08	0:38:07	0:58:24	1:02:55	1:19:12	1:23:49	2:56:53
780	0:18:26	0:30:19	0:38:21	0:58:47	1:03:19	1:19:42	1:24:22	2:58:01
775	0:18:34	0:30:31	0:38:36	0:59:10	1:03:43	1:20:13	1:24:54	2:59:10
770	0:18:41	0:30:43	0:38:51	0:59:33	1:04:08	1:20:44	1:25:27	3:00:19
765	0:18:48	0:30:55	0:39:06	0:59:56	1:04:33	1:21:16	1:26:01	3:01:30
760	0:18:56	0:31:07	0:39:22	1:00:20	1:04:59	1:21:48	1:26:35	3:02:42
755	0:19:03	0:31:19	0:39:37	1:00:44	1:05:25	1:22:20	1:27:09	3:03:54
750	0:19:11	0:31:32	0:39:53	1:01:08	1:05:51	1:22:53	1:27:44	3:05:08
745	0:19:18	0:31:45	0:40:09	1:01:33	1:06:17	1:23:27	1:28:19	3:06:23
740	0:19:26	0:31:58	0:40:26	1:01:58	1:06:44	1:24:01	1:28:55	3:07:38
735	0:19:34	0:32:11	0:40:42	1:02:23	1:07:11	1:24:35	1:29:31	3:08:55
730	0:19:42	0:32:24	0:40:59	1:02:48	1:07:39	1:25:10	1:30:08	3:10:12
725	0:19:50	0:32:37	0:41:16	1:03:14	1:08:07	1:25:45	1:30:46	3:11:31
720	0:19:59	0:32:51	0:41:33	1:03:41	1:08:35	1:26:21	1:31:23	3:12:51
715	0:20:07	0:33:05	0:41:50	1:04:08	1:09:04	1:26:57	1:32:02	3:14:12
710	0:20:15	0:33:19	0:42:08	1:04:35	1:09:33	1:27:34	1:32:41	3:15:34
705	0:20:24	0:33:33	0:42:26	1:05:02	1:10:03	1:28:11	1:33:20	3:16:57
700	0:20:33	0:33:47	0:42:44	1:05:30	1:10:33	1:28:49	1:34:00	3:18:21
695	0:20:42	0:34:02	0:43:03	1:05:58	1:11:03	1:29:27	1:34:41	3:19:47
690	0:20:51	0:34:17	0:43:21	1:06:27	1:11:34	1:30:06	1:35:22	3:21:14
685	0:21:00	0:34:32	0:43:40	1:06:56	1:12:06	1:30:45	1:36:04	3:22:42
680	0:21:09	0:34:47	0:44:00	1:07:26	1:12:37	1:31:25	1:36:46	3:24:11
675	0:21:19	0:35:02	0:44:19	1:07:56	1:13:10	1:32:06	1:37:29	3:25:42
670	0:21:28	0:35:18	0:44:39	1:08:26	1:13:42	1:32:47	1:38:13	3:27:14
665	0:21:38	0:35:34	0:44:59	1:08:57	1:14:16	1:33:29	1:38:57	3:28:48
660	0:21:48	0:35:50	0:45:20	1:09:28	1:14:49	1:34:12	1:39:42	3:30:23
655	0:21:58	0:36:06	0:45:40	1:10:00	1:15:24	1:34:55	1:40:27	3:31:59
650	0:22:08	0:36:23	0:46:02	1:10:32	1:15:58	1:35:38	1:41:14	3:33:37
645	0:22:18	0:36:40	0:46:23	1:11:05	1:16:34	1:36:23	1:42:01	3:35:16
640	0:22:28	0:36:57	0:46:45	1:11:38	1:17:10	1:37:08	1:42:49	3:36:57

RATING	5K	8K/5M	10K	15K	10M	20K	1/2 Marathon	Marathon
635	0:22:39	0:37:15	0:47:07	1:12:12	1:17:46	1:37:54	1:43:37	3:38:40
630	0:22:50	0:37:32	0:47:29	1:12:47	1:18:23	1:38:41	1:44:27	3:40:24
625	0:23:01	0:37:50	0:47:52	1:13:22	1:19:01	1:39:28	1:45:17	3:42:10
620	0:23:12	0:38:09	0:48:15	1:13:57	1:19:39	1:40:16	1:46:08	3:43:57
615	0:23:23	0:38:27	0:48:39	1:14:33	1:20:18	1:41:05	1:47:00	3:45:46
610	0:23:35	0:38:46	0:49:03	1:15:10	1:20:57	1:41:55	1:47:52	3:47:37
605	0:23:46	0:39:05	0:49:27	1:15:47	1:21:38	1:42:45	1:48:46	3:49:30
600	0:23:58	0:39:25	0:49:52	1:16:25	1:22:18	1:43:37	1:49:40	3:51:25
595	0:24:10	0:39:45	0:50:17	1:17:04	1:23:00	1:44:29	1:50:35	3:53:22
590	0:24:23	0:40:05	0:50:42	1:17:43	1:23:42	1:45:22	1:51:32	3:55:20
585	0:24:35	0:40:26	0:51:08	1:18:23	1:24:25	1:46:16	1:52:29	3:57:21
580	0:24:48	0:40:47	0:51:35	1:19:03	1:25:09	1:47:11	1:53:27	3:59:24
575	0:25:01	0:41:08	0:52:02	1:19:44	1:25:53	1:48:07	1:54:26	4:01:29
570	0:25:14	0:41:29	0:52:29	1:20:26	1:26:38	1:49:04	1:55:26	4:03:36
565	0:25:27	0:41:52	0:52:57	1:21:09	1:27:24	1:50:02	1:56:28	4:05:45
560	0:25:41	0:42:14	0:53:25	1:21:52	1:28:11	1:51:01	1:57:30	4:07:57
555	0:25:55	0:42:37	0:53:54	1:22:37	1:28:59	1:52:01	1:58:34	4:10:11
550	0:26:09	0:43:00	0:54:24	1:23:22	1:29:47	1:53:02	1:59:38	4:12:27
545	0:26:23	0:43:24	0:54:54	1:24:08	1:30:37	1:54:04	2:00:44	4:14:46
540	0:26:38	0:43:48	0:55:24	1:24:54	1:31:27	1:55:07	2:01:51	4:17:08
535	0:26:53	0:44:12	0:55:55	1:25:42	1:32:18	1:56:12	2:02:59	4:19:32
530	0:27:08	0:44:37	0:56:27	1:26:31	1:33:11	1:57:18	2:04:09	4:21:59
525	0:27:24	0:45:03	0:56:59	1:27:20	1:34:04	1:58:25	2:05:20	4:24:29
520	0:27:40	0:45:29	0:57:32	1:28:10	1:34:58	1:59:33	2:06:32	4:27:01
515	0:27:56	0:45:55	0:58:05	1:29:02	1:35:53	2:00:43	2:07:46	4:29:37
510	0:28:12	0:46:22	0:58:40	1:29:54	1:36:50	2:01:54	2:09:01	4:32:15
505	0:28:29	0:46:50	0:59:14	1:30:48	1:37:47	2:03:06	2:10:18	4:34:57
500	0:28:46	0:47:18	0:59:50	1:31:42	1:38:46	2:04:20	2:11:36	4:37:42
495	0:29:03	0:47:47	1:00:26	1:32:38	1:39:46	2:05:35	2:12:56	4:40:30
490	0:29:21	0:48:16	1:01:03	1:33:34	1:40:47	2:06:52	2:14:17	4:43:22
485	0:29:39	0:48:46	1:01:41	1:34:32	1:41:49	2:08:11	2:15:40	4:46:17
480	0:29:58	0:49:16	1:02:20	1:35:31	1:42:53	2:09:31	2:17:05	4:49:16
475	0:30:17	0:49:47	1:02:59	1:36:32	1:43:58	2:10:53	2:18:32	4:52:19
470	0:30:36	0:50:19	1:03:39	1:37:33	1:45:04	2:12:16	2:20:00	4:55:26
465	0:30:56	0:50:52	1:04:20	1:38:36	1:46:12	2:13:42	2:21:30	4:58:36
460	0:31:16	0:51:25	1:05:02	1:39:40	1:47:21	2:15:09	2:23:03	5:01:51
455	0:31:37	0:51:59	1:05:45	1:40:46	1:48:32	2:16:38	2:24:37	5:05:10
450	0:31:58	0:52:33	1:06:29	1:41:53	1:49:44	2:18:09	2:26:13	5:08:33
445	0:32:19	0:53:09	1:07:14	1:43:02	1:50:58	2:19:42	2:27:52	5:12:01
440	0:32:41	0:53:45	1:08:00	1:44:12	1:52:14	2:21:17	2:29:33	5:15:34
435	0:33:04	0:54:22	1:08:46	1:45:24	1:53:31	2:22:55	2:31:16	5:19:12
430	0:33:27	0:55:00	1:09:34	1:46:38	1:54:51	2:24:34	2:33:01	5:22:54
425	0:33:51	0:55:39	1:10:24	1:47:53	1:56:12	2:26:16	2:34:49	5:26:42
420	0:34:15	0:56:19	1:11:14	1:49:10	1:57:35	2:28:01	2:36:40	5:30:36
415	0:34:40	0:56:59	1:12:05	1:50:29	1:59:00	2:29:48	2:38:33	5:34:35
410	0:35:05	0:57:41	1:12:58	1:51:50	2:00:27	2:31:38	2:40:29	5:38:40
405	0:35:31	0:58:24	1:13:52	1:53:13	2:01:56	2:33:30	2:42:28	5:42:50
400	0:35:58	0:59:07	1:14:48	1:54:37	2:03:28	2:35:25	2:44:30	5:47:08
395	0:36:25	0:59:52	1:15:44	1:56:05	2:05:01	2:37:23	2:46:35	5:51:31
390	0:36:53	1:00:38	1:16:43	1:57:34	2:06:37	2:39:24	2:48:43	5:56:02
385	0:37:22	1:01:26	1:17:42	1:59:05	2:08:16	2:41:28	2:50:55	6:00:39
380	0:37:51	1:02:14	1:18:44	2:00:39	2:09:57	2:43:36	2:53:09	6:05:24
375	0:38:21	1:03:04	1:19:47	2:02:16	2:11:41	2:45:47	2:55:28	6:10:16

Age-Adjusted and Age-Graded
Race Time Charts

Our best performance years as runners come somewhere between ages 20 and 34. You may run your fastest times after those years, but most likely this is because you didn't train and race as seriously when you were younger. To help keep runners motivated as race times slow with age, most races offer awards in 5- or 10-year age groups starting at age 35 or 40. But masters runners of all levels can be motivated by the age-graded scoring tables developed by the World Association of Veteran Athletes (WAVA). Indeed, I used them as a goal when I made my comeback as a 50-year-old. It was motivating to be able to run times that were the age-adjusted equal to my prime twenty years earlier and to aim for national-class times.

To help you do this, we've provided two charts: Age-adjusted, which converts your race performances to what you theoretically could have run in your prime years; and Age-graded, which converts your race times to a percentage of the standard for your age. The latter will give you a rating score for comparison with other race distances (and to other runners of all ages). The complete charts for ages 8 to 100 for road racing and track-and-field events can be ordered from National Masters News, P.O. Box 16597, North Hollywood, CA 91615-6597.

THE AGE-ADJUSTED CHART

The age factors on this chart express the rate of decline based on age as compared with the world record by an open-class runner (age 20 to 34). To determine your age-adjusted time for a race:

1. *Convert your race time to seconds* by multiplying the minutes by 60 and adding this total to the leftover seconds:

    The sample is a 53-year-old woman with a 10K time of 45:18.

    45:18 = (45 minutes × 60) + (18 seconds)

    45:18 = 2,700 seconds + 18 seconds = 2,718 seconds

2. *Multiply this time by the age factor* for the specific race distance, age, and gender:

    The age factor for a 53-year-old woman for 10K is .8545 (see chart).

    2,718 seconds × .8545 = 2,323 seconds

3. *Convert this time to minutes:seconds:*

    2,323 seconds divided by 60 seconds = 38.72 minutes

    .72 minute × 60 seconds = 43 seconds

    2,323 seconds = 38:43 (38 minutes and 43 seconds)

Thus, this runner's time of 45:18 is equal to her potential prime-age time of 38:43.

I was thrilled to run 18:45 for 5K as I turned 50 while finishing this diary. It doesn't sound as good compared with my all-time best of 16:20 until I correct for age and get the adjusted time of 16:45. So I really didn't get too much older or slower after all!

THE AGE-GRADED CHART

The time standards on this chart correspond approximately to world record marks for a person of that age and sex for each race distance when this table was compiled. The open-class (age 20 to 34) times are the overall world records (100 percent). You can use your performance-level percentage as a rating to compare to your scores at various distances, your scores from years past, your progress over the racing season, and to other runners—regardless of age or sex. Several races now use this scoring system to award the top performances in the race, regardless of age.

To determine your age-graded score for a race:

1. *Convert your race time to seconds* by multiplying the minutes by 60 and adding to the leftover seconds.

    Again, the sample is a 53-year-old woman with a 10K time of 45:18.

$45:18 = (45 \text{ minutes} \times 60) + (18 \text{ seconds})$
$45:18 = 2,700 \text{ seconds} + 18 \text{ seconds} = 2,718 \text{ seconds}$

2. *Convert the single-age standard time for your sex to seconds:*
   Age 53 female standard for 10K = 35:00
   $35:00 = 35 \text{ minutes} \times 60 = 2,100 \text{ seconds}$

3. *Divide the standard race time for the specific race distance by your race time.*
   2,100 seconds divided by 2,718 seconds = .77 = 77 percent

Thus, her performance-level percentage score is 77 percent. Note this score for each of your races in the rating column on the Record of Races chart on page 126 and the Personal Records chart on page 128. My age 50 time of 18:45 for 5K (compared with the age 50 standard of 14:31.6) resulted in a score of 77 percent. My challenging goal is to reach the national class standard of 80 percent.

How do you rate compared with the big guns? Here's the WAVA Achievement levels:

100%	Approximate World-Record Level
Over 90%	World-Class Level
Over 80%	National-Class Level
Over 70%	Regional-Class Level
Over 60%	Local-Class Level

AGE-ADJUSTED RACE TIME FACTORS (MEN)

AGE	5K	5 MILE/8K	10K	15K	10 MILE	20K	½ MAR	MAR
20–34	1.0000	1.0000	1.0000	1.0000	1.0000	1.0000	1.0000	1.0000
35	0.9963	1.0000	1.0000	1.0000	1.0000	1.0000	1.0000	1.0000
36	0.9895	0.9934	0.9953	0.9989	0.9996	1.0000	1.0000	1.0000
37	0.9827	0.9866	0.9884	0.9921	0.9928	0.9951	0.9957	1.0000
38	0.9760	0.9797	0.9816	0.9852	0.9859	0.9882	0.9888	0.9973
39	0.9692	0.9729	0.9747	0.9784	0.9791	0.9814	0.9820	0.9904
40	0.9624	0.9661	0.9679	0.9715	0.9722	0.9745	0.9751	0.9835
41	0.9555	0.9592	0.9610	0.9646	0.9653	0.9676	0.9682	0.9765
42	0.9487	0.9523	0.9541	0.9576	0.9583	0.9606	0.9612	0.9695
43	0.9418	0.9454	0.9471	0.9507	0.9514	0.9537	0.9543	0.9626
44	0.9350	0.9385	0.9402	0.9437	0.9444	0.9467	0.9473	0.9556
45	0.9281	0.9316	0.9333	0.9368	0.9375	0.9398	0.9404	0.9486
46	0.9211	0.9246	0.9262	0.9297	0.9304	0.9327	0.9333	0.9415
47	0.9141	0.9175	0.9192	0.9226	0.9233	0.9256	0.9262	0.9344
48	0.9071	0.9105	0.9121	0.9156	0.9163	0.9186	0.9192	0.9272
49	0.9001	0.9034	0.9051	0.9085	0.9092	0.9115	0.9121	0.9201
50	0.8931	0.8964	0.8980	0.9014	0.9021	0.9044	0.9050	0.9130
51	0.8859	0.8891	0.8907	0.8941	0.8948	0.8971	0.8977	0.9057
52	0.8787	0.8819	0.8834	0.8868	0.8875	0.8898	0.8904	0.8983
53	0.8714	0.8746	0.8762	0.8795	0.8802	0.8825	0.8831	0.8910
54	0.8642	0.8674	0.8689	0.8722	0.8729	0.8752	0.8758	0.8836
55	0.8570	0.8601	0.8616	0.8649	0.8656	0.8679	0.8685	0.8763
56	0.8495	0.8525	0.8540	0.8573	0.8580	0.8603	0.8609	0.8686
57	0.8419	0.8449	0.8464	0.8497	0.8504	0.8527	0.8533	0.8610
58	0.8344	0.8374	0.8388	0.8420	0.8427	0.8450	0.8456	0.8533
59	0.8268	0.8298	0.8312	0.8344	0.8351	0.8374	0.8380	0.8457
60	0.8193	0.8222	0.8236	0.8268	0.8275	0.8298	0.8304	0.8380
61	0.8113	0.8142	0.8156	0.8187	0.8194	0.8217	0.8223	0.8299
62	0.8033	0.8062	0.8075	0.8107	0.8114	0.8137	0.8143	0.8218
63	0.7954	0.7981	0.7995	0.8026	0.8033	0.8056	0.8062	0.8137
64	0.7874	0.7901	0.7914	0.7946	0.7953	0.7976	0.7982	0.8056
65	0.7794	0.7821	0.7834	0.7865	0.7872	0.7895	0.7901	0.7975
66	0.7708	0.7735	0.7748	0.7779	0.7786	0.7809	0.7815	0.7888
67	0.7623	0.7649	0.7662	0.7692	0.7699	0.7722	0.7728	0.7801
68	0.7537	0.7563	0.7575	0.7606	0.7613	0.7636	0.7642	0.7715
69	0.7452	0.7477	0.7489	0.7519	0.7526	0.7549	0.7555	0.7628
70	0.7366	0.7391	0.7403	0.7433	0.7440	0.7463	0.7469	0.7541
71	0.7273	0.7298	0.7309	0.7339	0.7346	0.7369	0.7375	0.7447
72	0.7180	0.7204	0.7216	0.7245	0.7252	0.7275	0.7281	0.7353
73	0.7087	0.7111	0.7122	0.7152	0.7159	0.7182	0.7188	0.7258
74	0.6994	0.7017	0.7029	0.7058	0.7065	0.7088	0.7094	0.7164
75	0.6901	0.6924	0.6935	0.6964	0.6971	0.6994	0.7000	0.7070
76	0.6798	0.6821	0.6832	0.6861	0.6868	0.6891	0.6897	0.6966
77	0.6696	0.6718	0.6729	0.6757	0.6764	0.6787	0.6793	0.6862
78	0.6593	0.6615	0.6625	0.6654	0.6661	0.6684	0.6690	0.6759
79	0.6491	0.6512	0.6522	0.6550	0.6557	0.6580	0.6586	0.6655
80	0.6388	0.6409	0.6419	0.6447	0.6454	0.6477	0.6483	0.6551
85	0.5807	0.5826	0.5835	0.5862	0.5869	0.5892	0.5898	0.5964
90	0.5111	0.5128	0.5136	0.5162	0.5169	0.5192	0.5198	0.5262
95	0.4172	0.4187	0.4194	0.4219	0.4226	0.4249	0.4255	0.4317
100	0.2619	0.2632	0.2638	0.2662	0.2669	0.2692	0.2698	0.2758

AGE-ADJUSTED RACE TIME FACTORS (WOMEN)

AGE	5K	5 MILE/8K	10K	15K	10 MILE	20K	½ MAR	MAR
20–34	1.0000	1.0000	1.0000	1.0000	1.0000	1.0000	1.0000	1.0000
35	0.9913	0.9954	0.9974	1.0000	1.0000	1.0000	1.0000	1.0000
36	0.9835	0.9876	0.9896	0.9934	0.9941	0.9963	0.9969	1.0000
37	0.9758	0.9798	0.9818	0.9856	0.9863	0.9885	0.9891	0.9979
38	0.9680	0.9721	0.9741	0.9779	0.9786	0.9807	0.9813	0.9901
39	0.9603	0.9643	0.9663	0.9701	0.9708	0.9729	0.9735	0.9823
40	0.9525	0.9565	0.9585	0.9623	0.9630	0.9651	0.9657	0.9745
41	0.9447	0.9486	0.9506	0.9544	0.9551	0.9572	0.9578	0.9666
42	0.9368	0.9408	0.9428	0.9466	0.9473	0.9493	0.9499	0.9587
43	0.9290	0.9329	0.9349	0.9387	0.9394	0.9415	0.9421	0.9509
44	0.9211	0.9251	0.9271	0.9309	0.9316	0.9336	0.9342	0.9430
45	0.9133	0.9172	0.9192	0.9230	0.9237	0.9257	0.9263	0.9351
46	0.9053	0.9092	0.9112	0.9150	0.9157	0.9177	0.9183	0.9271
47	0.8973	0.9012	0.9032	0.9070	0.9077	0.9097	0.9103	0.9191
48	0.8894	0.8932	0.8952	0.8990	0.8997	0.9016	0.9022	0.9110
49	0.8814	0.8852	0.8872	0.8910	0.8917	0.8936	0.8942	0.9030
50	0.8734	0.8772	0.8792	0.8830	0.8837	0.8856	0.8862	0.8950
51	0.8652	0.8690	0.8710	0.8748	0.8755	0.8774	0.8780	0.8868
52	0.8570	0.8608	0.8628	0.8666	0.8673	0.8691	0.8697	0.8785
53	0.8488	0.8525	0.8545	0.8583	0.8590	0.8609	0.8615	0.8703
54	0.8406	0.8443	0.8463	0.8501	0.8508	0.8526	0.8532	0.8620
55	0.8324	0.8361	0.8381	0.8419	0.8426	0.8444	0.8450	0.8538
56	0.8239	0.8276	0.8296	0.8334	0.8341	0.8358	0.8364	0.8452
57	0.8154	0.8190	0.8210	0.8248	0.8255	0.8273	0.8279	0.8367
58	0.8068	0.8105	0.8125	0.8163	0.8170	0.8187	0.8193	0.8281
59	0.7983	0.8019	0.8039	0.8077	0.8084	0.8102	0.8108	0.8196
60	0.7898	0.7934	0.7954	0.7992	0.7999	0.8016	0.8022	0.8110
61	0.7808	0.7844	0.7864	0.7902	0.7909	0.7926	0.7932	0.8020
62	0.7719	0.7754	0.7774	0.7812	0.7819	0.7836	0.7842	0.7930
63	0.7629	0.7665	0.7685	0.7723	0.7730	0.7746	0.7752	0.7840
64	0.7540	0.7575	0.7595	0.7633	0.7640	0.7656	0.7662	0.7750
65	0.7450	0.7485	0.7505	0.7543	0.7550	0.7566	0.7572	0.7660
66	0.7355	0.7389	0.7409	0.7447	0.7454	0.7470	0.7476	0.7564
67	0.7259	0.7294	0.7314	0.7352	0.7359	0.7374	0.7380	0.7468
68	0.7164	0.7198	0.7218	0.7256	0.7263	0.7279	0.7285	0.7373
69	0.7068	0.7103	0.7123	0.7161	0.7168	0.7183	0.7189	0.7277
70	0.6973	0.7007	0.7027	0.7065	0.7072	0.7087	0.7093	0.7181
71	0.6870	0.6904	0.6924	0.6962	0.6969	0.6984	0.6990	0.7078
72	0.6767	0.6801	0.6821	0.6859	0.6866	0.6881	0.6887	0.6975
73	0.6665	0.6698	0.6718	0.6756	0.6763	0.6777	0.6783	0.6871
74	0.6562	0.6595	0.6615	0.6653	0.6660	0.6674	0.6680	0.6768
75	0.6459	0.6492	0.6512	0.6550	0.6557	0.6571	0.6577	0.6665
76	0.6347	0.6379	0.6399	0.6437	0.6444	0.6458	0.6464	0.6552
77	0.6234	0.6267	0.6287	0.6325	0.6332	0.6345	0.6351	0.6439
78	0.6122	0.6154	0.6174	0.6212	0.6219	0.6233	0.6239	0.6327
79	0.6009	0.6042	0.6062	0.6100	0.6107	0.6120	0.6126	0.6214
80	0.5897	0.5929	0.5949	0.5987	0.5994	0.6007	0.6013	0.6101
85	0.5267	0.5298	0.5318	0.5356	0.5363	0.5375	0.5381	0.5469
90	0.4522	0.4552	0.4572	0.4610	0.4617	0.4628	0.4634	0.4722
95	0.3534	0.3563	0.3583	0.3621	0.3628	0.3638	0.3644	0.3732
100	0.1932	0.1960	0.1980	0.2018	0.2025	0.2034	0.2040	0.2128

AGE-GRADED RACE TIME STANDARDS (MEN)

AGE	5K	5 MILE/8K	10K	15K	10 MILE	20K	½ MAR	MAR
20–34	12:58.4	21:18.9	26:58.4	41:26	44:40	56:20	59:39	2:06:50
35	13:01.3	21:18.9	26:58.4	41:26	44:40	56:20	59:39	2:06:50
36	13:06.6	21:27.4	27:06.1	41:29	44:41	56:20	59:39	2:06:50
37	13:12.1	21:36.3	27:17.3	41:46	44:59	56:37	0:59:55	2:06:50
38	13:17.6	21:45.3	27:28.7	42:03	45:18	57:00	1:00:19	2:07:11
39	13:23.1	21:54.5	27:40.3	42:21	45:37	57:24	1:00:45	2:08:04
40	13:28.8	22:03.7	27:52.1	42:39	45:57	57:48	1:01:10	2:08:58
41	13:34.6	22:13.3	28:04.1	42:57	46:16	58:13	1:01:37	2:09:53
42	13:40.5	22:22.9	28:16.3	43:16	46:37	58:39	1:02:03	2:10:49
43	13:46.5	22:32.7	28:28.7	43:35	46:57	59:04	1:02:30	2:11:46
44	13:52.5	22:42.7	28:41.3	43:54	47:18	59:30	1:02:58	2:12:44
45	13:58.7	22:52.8	28:54.0	44:14	47:39	59:57	1:03:26	2:13:42
46	14:05.1	23:03.2	29:07.3	44:34	48:00	1:00:24	1:03:55	2:14:43
47	14:11.5	23:13.8	29:20.7	44:54	48:23	1:00:52	1:04:24	2:15:45
48	14:18.1	23:24.6	29:34.3	45:15	48:45	1:01:20	1:04:54	2:16:47
49	14:24.8	23:35.6	29:48.1	45:36	49:08	1:01:48	1:05:24	2:17:51
50	14:31.6	23:46.7	30:02.2	45:58	49:31	1:02:17	1:05:55	2:18:55
51	14:38.7	23:58.3	30:16.9	46:20	49:55	1:02:48	1:06:27	2:20:03
52	14:45.9	24:10.2	30:31.9	46:43	50:20	1:03:19	1:06:60	2:21:11
53	14:53.2	24:22.2	30:47.1	47:07	50:45	1:03:50	1:07:33	2:22:21
54	15:00.7	24:34.4	31:02.6	47:30	51:10	1:04:22	1:08:07	2:23:32
55	15:08.3	24:46.9	31:18.3	47:54	51:36	1:04:54	1:08:41	2:24:44
56	15:16.3	25:00.1	31:35.1	48:20	52:04	1:05:29	1:09:17	2:26:01
57	15:24.5	25:13.6	31:52.1	48:46	52:32	1:06:04	1:09:55	2:27:19
58	15:32.9	25:27.3	32:09.4	49:12	53:00	1:06:40	1:10:32	2:28:38
59	15:41.4	25:41.2	32:27.0	49:39	53:29	1:07:16	1:11:11	2:29:59
60	15:50.1	25:55.4	32:45.0	50:07	53:59	1:07:53	1:11:50	2:31:21
61	15:59.4	26:10.7	33:04.4	50:36	54:31	1:08:33	1:12:32	2:32:50
62	16:08.9	26:26.4	33:24.1	51:07	55:03	1:09:14	1:13:15	2:34:20
63	16:18.7	26:42.3	33:44.3	51:37	55:36	1:09:56	1:13:69	2:35:52
64	16:28.6	26:58.6	34:04.9	52:09	56:10	1:10:38	1:14:44	2:37:26
65	16:38.7	27:15.2	34:25.8	52:41	56:44	1:11:21	1:15:30	2:39:02
66	16:49.8	27:33.4	34:48.8	53:16	57:22	1:12:09	1:16:20	2:40:47
67	17:01.1	27:51.9	35:12.3	53:52	58:01	1:12:57	1:17:11	2:42:35
68	17:12.7	28:11.0	35:36.4	54:29	58:40	1:13:47	1:18:03	2:44:24
69	17:24.6	28:30.4	36:01.0	55:06	59:21	1:14:37	1:18:57	2:46:17
70	17:36.7	28:50.3	36:26.1	55:45	1:00:02	1:15:29	1:19:52	2:48:11
71	17:50.2	29:12.5	36:54.1	56:27	1:00:48	1:16:27	1:20:53	2:50:19
72	18:04.1	29:35.2	37:22.8	57:11	1:01:35	1:17:26	1:21:55	2:52:30
73	18:18.3	29:58.5	37:52.3	57:56	1:02:24	1:18:26	1:22:59	2:54:44
74	18:32.9	30:22.4	38:22.6	58:42	1:03:13	1:19:29	1:24:05	2:57:02
75	18:47.9	30:47.0	38:53.6	59:30	1:04:04	1:20:33	1:25:13	2:59:24
76	19:05.0	31:14.9	39:28.9	1:00:24	1:05:02	1:21:45	1:26:30	3:02:04
77	19:22.5	31:43.6	40:05.2	1:01:19	1:06:02	1:22:60	1:27:49	3:04:49
78	19:40.6	32:13.3	40:42.7	1:02:16	1:07:04	1:24:17	1:29:10	3:07:40
79	19:59.3	32:43.9	41:21.3	1:03:15	1:08:07	1:25:36	1:30:34	3:10:35
80	20:18.5	33:15.4	42:01.2	1:04:16	1:09:12	1:26:58	1:32:01	3:13:37
85	22:20.4	36:35.1	46:13.6	1:10:41	1:16:06	1:35:37	1:41:08	3:32:40
90	25:23.0	41:33.9	52:31.1	1:20:16	1:26:25	1:48:30	1:54:45	4:01:02
95	31:05.7	50:54.4	1:04:19	1:38:12	1:45:42	2:12:35	2:20:11	4:53:48
100	49:32.1	1:20:59	1:42:15	2:35:39	2:47:21	3:29:16	3:41:05	7:39:52

AGE-GRADED RACE TIME STANDARD (WOMEN)

AGE	5K	5 MILE/8K	10K	15K	10 MILE	20K	½ MAR	MAR
20–34	14:23.7	23:39.0	29:55.0	45:51	49:23	1:02:10	1:05:48	2:18:51
35	14:31.3	23:45.6	29:59.7	45:51	49:23	1:02:10	1:05:48	2:18:51
36	14:38.1	23:56.8	30:13.8	46:09	49:41	1:02:24	1:06:00	2:18:51
37	14:45.1	24:08.2	30:28.2	46:31	50:04	1:02:53	1:06:32	2:19:09
38	14:52.2	24:19.8	30:42.8	46:53	50:28	1:03:23	1:07:03	2:20:14
39	14:59.4	24:31.6	30:57.6	47:16	50:52	1:03:54	1:07:35	2:21:21
40	15:06.8	24:43.5	31:12.7	47:39	51:17	1:04:25	1:08:08	2:22:29
41	15:14.3	24:55.8	31:28.2	48:02	51:42	1:04:57	1:08:42	2:23:39
42	15:21.9	25:08.3	31:43.9	48:26	52:08	1:05:29	1:09:16	2:24:50
43	15:29.7	25:21.0	31:60.0	48:51	52:34	1:06:02	1:09:51	2:26:02
44	15:37.6	25:34.0	32:16.2	49:15	53:01	1:06:35	1:10:26	2:27:15
45	15:45.7	25:47.1	32:32.8	49:40	53:28	1:07:09	1:11:02	2:28:29
46	15:54.0	26:00.7	32:49.9	50:07	53:56	1:07:45	1:11:39	2:29:46
47	16:02.5	26:14.6	33:07.4	50:33	54:24	1:08:20	1:12:17	2:31:05
48	16:11.1	26:28.7	33:25.1	51:00	54:53	1:08:57	1:12:56	2:32:24
49	16:19.9	26:43.0	33:43.2	51:28	55:23	1:09:34	1:13:35	2:33:46
50	16:28.9	26:57.6	34:01.6	51:56	55:53	1:10:12	1:14:15	2:35:08
51	16:38.3	27:12.9	34:20.9	52:25	56:24	1:10:51	1:14:57	2:36:35
52	16:47.8	27:28.5	34:40.5	52:55	56:57	1:11:32	1:15:39	2:38:03
53	16:57.5	27:44.4	35:00.5	53:25	57:29	1:12:13	1:16:23	2:39:33
54	17:07.5	28:00.6	35:20.9	53:56	58:03	1:12:55	1:17:07	2:41:04
55	17:17.6	28:17.2	35:41.7	54:28	58:36	1:13:37	1:17:52	2:42:38
56	17:28.3	28:34.7	36:03.8	55:01	59:13	1:14:23	1:18:40	2:44:16
57	17:39.3	28:52.6	36:26.3	55:35	59:49	1:15:09	1:19:29	2:45:57
58	17:50.5	29:10.8	36:49.3	56:10	1:00:27	1:15:56	1:20:19	2:47:40
59	18:01.9	29:29.5	37:12.8	56:46	1:01:05	1:16:44	1:21:10	2:49:25
60	18:13.6	29:48.5	37:36.7	57:22	1:01:44	1:17:33	1:22:01	2:51:13
61	18:26.1	30:09.0	38:02.5	58:01	1:02:26	1:18:26	1:22:57	2:53:08
62	18:38.9	30:29.9	38:28.9	58:41	1:03:09	1:19:20	1:23:54	2:55:06
63	18:52.1	30:51.4	38:55.8	59:22	1:03:53	1:20:15	1:24:53	2:57:06
64	19:05.5	31:13.3	39:23.5	1:00:04	1:04:38	1:21:12	1:25:53	2:59:10
65	19:19.3	31:35.8	39:51.7	1:00:47	1:05:25	1:22:10	1:26:50	3:01:16
66	19:34.4	32:00.3	40:22.6	1:01:34	1:06:15	1:23:13	1:28:01	3:03:34
67	19:49.8	32:25.5	40:54.3	1:02:22	1:07:06	1:24:18	1:29:09	3:05:55
68	20:05.6	32:51.3	41:26.8	1:03:11	1:07:59	1:25:25	1:30:20	3:08:20
69	20:21.9	33:17.9	42:00.1	1:04:02	1:08:54	·1:26:33	1:31:32	3:10:49
70	20:38.6	33:45.1	42:34.4	1:04:54	1:09:50	1:27:43	1:32:46	3:13:21
71	20:57.2	34:15.3	43:12.4	1:05:51	1:10:52	1:29:01	1:34:08	3:16:11
72	21:16.3	34:46.5	43:51.6	1:06:51	1:11:55	1:30:21	1:35:33	3:19:05
73	21:35.9	35:18.5	44:31.9	1:07:52	1:13:01	1:31:44	1:37:00	3:22:04
74	21:56.2	35:51.6	45:13.5	1:08:55	1:14:09	1:33:09	1:38:30	3:25:09
75	22:17.2	36:25.8	45:56.4	1:10:00	1:15:19	1:34:36	1:40:03	3:28:20
76	22:40.9	37:04.3	46:45.0	1:11:13	1:16:38	1:36:16	1:41:47	3:31:55
77	23:05.4	37:44.3	47:35.2	1:12:30	1:17:60	1:37:58	1:43:36	3:35:38
78	23:30.8	38:25.7	48:27.3	1:13:48	1:19:24	1:39:45	1:45:28	3:39:28
79	23:57.2	39:08.7	49:21.3	1:15:10	1:20:52	1:41:35	1:47:25	3:43:27
80	24:24.6	39:53.3	50:17.3	1:16:35	1:22:23	1:43:29	1:49:26	3:47:35
85	27:19.8	44:38.4	56:15.3	1:25:36	1:32:05	1:55:40	2:02:17	4:13:53
90	31:50.0	51:57.3	1:05:26	1:39:27	1:46:58	2:14:20	2:21:60	4:54:03
95	40:43.9	1:06:23	1:23:30	2:06:37	2:16:07	2:50:53	3:00:34	6:12:03
100	1:14:30	2:00:40	2:31:06	3:47:12	4:03:52	5:05:38	5:22:33	10:52:29

PART III

Training

Introduction to Training Schedules
for All Levels

The following training schedules are from *The Runner's Handbook* and *The Competitive Runner's Handbook* and are the official training programs for the New York Road Runners Club classes. Thousands of runners each year successfully follow these recommended programs.

BEGINNER AND ADVANCED BEGINNER RUNNER

The Beginner Runner can walk briskly for at least 20 minutes, but can't comfortably run a full mile. The goal for this runner is to build up to running for 20 minutes nonstop. The Advanced Beginner Runner can comfortably run one mile nonstop. The goal for this runner is to build up to running for 30 minutes nonstop.

Begin the enclosed build-up schedule at the level you can comfortably handle. If you have been sedentary and are just starting a running program, start at week 1 of the Beginner schedule. If you are fairly active and can already run a mile or so—or at least for ten minutes—then start with the Advanced Beginner program. Run the recommended workout at least three times per week (preferably five) before moving up to the next week's schedule. Most runners benefit from following the schedules exactly. If you can't keep up with the progression, repeat the week's program until you feel comfortable. If you find the program too easy, simply adjust by moving up to a week that is more challenging but not too difficult. Continue from there. Be cautious, it is better to start at too low a level and work up gradually than to start too high and struggle. Consult *The Runner's Handbook* for detailed training guidelines for the Beginner and Advanced Beginner Runner.

INTERMEDIATE RUNNER/NOVICE COMPETITOR, BASIC COMPETITOR, COMPETITOR, AND ADVANCED COMPETITOR

Use the enclosed sample build-up schedules for the following general categories of runners to help you run stronger, longer, and faster:

- The Intermediate Runner/Novice Competitor can run at least 30 minutes nonstop and races 5K–10K distances slower than 9 minutes per mile.

- The Basic Competitor races 5K–10K distances at approximately 8–9 minutes per mile.

- The Competitor races at 5K–10K distances approximately 7–8 minutes per mile.

- The Advanced Competitor races 5K–10K distances at faster than 7 minutes per mile.

The schedules start with a base week that you should hold for at least 3–4 weeks before moving up. Begin with a comfortable level and gradually increase mileage following the sample schedule. Level off when you meet your goal. Refer to the chart of recommended mileage for various race distances on page 156. These are *sample* schedules that will give you a good base for racing 5K–½ marathon distances. Adapt them to fit your personal needs. Use the daily mileage recommendations as a guide. Consult *The Competitive Runner's Handbook* for detailed training guidelines for the specific racing distances of one mile, 5K, 10K, and ½ marathon.

SAMPLE 10-WEEK BEGINNER RUNNER'S TRAINING SCHEDULE

WEEK	RUN-WALK RATIO (MINUTES)	TOTAL RUN TIME
1	Run 1, walk 2. Complete sequence 7 times.	7
2	Run 2, walk 2. Complete sequence 5 times.	10
3	Run 3, walk 2. Complete sequence 4 times.	12
4	Run 5, walk 2. Complete sequence 3 times.	15
5	Run 6, walk 1½. Complete sequence 3 times.	18
6	Run 8, walk 1½. Complete sequence 2 times.	16
7	Run 10, walk 1½. Complete sequence 2 times.	20
8	Run 12, walk 1, run 8.	20
9	Run 15, walk 1, run 5.	20
10	Run 20 minutes nonstop.	20

SAMPLE 10-WEEK ADVANCED BEGINNER RUNNER'S TRAINING SCHEDULE

WEEK	RUN-WALK RATIO (MINUTES)	TOTAL RUN TIME
1	Run 10, walk 1½. Complete sequence 2 times.	20
2	Run 12, walk 1, run 8.	20
3	Run 15, walk 1, run 5.	20
4	Run 20 minutes nonstop.	20
5	Run 20 minutes nonstop.	20
6	Run 22 minutes nonstop.	22
7	Run 25 minutes nonstop.	25
8	Run 28 minutes nonstop.	28
9	Run 30 minutes nonstop.	30
10	Run 30 minutes nonstop.	30

NOTE: For both training programs above, warm up with 5–10 minutes of brisk walking. The run segments should be at a conversational pace, and walking segments should be at a brisk pace. Cool down with 5–10 minutes of slow walking.

SAMPLE 10-WEEK INTERMEDIATE RUNNER/NOVICE COMPETITOR TRAINING SCHEDULE: BUILDING FROM A 10-MILE-A-WEEK BASE TO 20 MILES

WEEKS	MON	TUES	WED	THUR	FRI	SAT	SUN	TOTAL
BASE	Off	3	Off	2	Off	3	2	10
1	Off	3	Off	3	Off	3	2	11
2	Off	3	Off	3	Off	3	3	12
3	Off	3	Off	3	Off	4	3	13
4	Off	3	Off	3	Off	4	3	13
5	Off	3	2	3	Off	4	3	15
6	Off	3	2	3	Off	4	3	15
7	Off	3	3	3	Off	5	3	17
8	Off	3	3	4	Off	5	3	18
9	Off	3	4	4	Off	5	3	19
10	Off	3	4	4	Off	6	3	20

SAMPLE 10-WEEK INTERMEDIATE RUNNER/NOVICE COMPETITOR TRAINING SCHEDULE: BUILDING FROM A 20-MILE-A-WEEK BASE TO 30 MILES

WEEKS	MON	TUES	WED	THUR	FRI	SAT	SUN	TOTAL
BASE	Off	3	4	4	Off	6	3	20
1	Off	3	4	4	Off	6	4	21
2	Off	3	4	4	Off	7	4	22
3	Off	3	4	4	Off	5	4	20
4	Off	3	4	4	Off	8	4	23
5	Off	3	4	5	Off	8	4	24
6	Off	3	4	5	Off	8	4	24
7	Off	3	5	5	Off	8	4	25
8	Off	3	4	4	Off	6	3	20
9	Off	3	4	5	3	8	4	27
10	Off	3	4	6	4	8	5	30

SAMPLE 10-WEEK BASIC COMPETITOR TRAINING SCHEDULE: BUILDING FROM A 20-MILE-A-WEEK BASE TO 30 MILES

WEEKS	MON	TUES	WED	THUR	FRI	SAT	SUN	TOTAL
BASE	Off	3	4	4	Off	6	3	20
1	Off	3	4	4	Off	6	4	21
2	Off	3	4	4	Off	7	4	22
3	Off	3	4	4	Off	5	4	20
4	Off	3	4	4	Off	8	4	23
5	Off	3	4	5	Off	8	4	24
6	Off	3	4	5	Off	8	4	24
7	Off	3	5	5	Off	8	4	25
8	Off	3	4	4	Off	6	3	20
9	Off	3	4	5	3	8	4	27
10	Off	3	4	6	4	8	5	30

SAMPLE 10-WEEK BASIC COMPETITOR TRAINING SCHEDULE: BUILDING FROM A 30-MILE-A-WEEK BASE TO 40 MILES

WEEKS	MON	TUES	WED	THUR	FRI	SAT	SUN	TOTAL
BASE	Off	3	4	6	4	8	5	30
1	Off	4	5	6	4	8	5	32
2	Off	4	5	6	4	10	5	34
3	Off	4	5	6	4	10	5	34
4	Off	3	4	6	4	8	5	30
5	Off	4	5	6	4	12	5	36
6	Off	4	5	6	4	12	5	36
7	Off	4	6	6	4	12	6	38
8	Off	3	4	6	4	8	5	30
9	Off	4	6	6	4	12	6	38
10	Off	4	6	6	6	12	6	40

SAMPLE 10-WEEK COMPETITOR TRAINING SCHEDULE: BUILDING FROM A 30-MILE-A-WEEK BASE TO 40 MILES

WEEKS	MON	TUES	WED	THUR	FRI	SAT	SUN	TOTAL
BASE	Off	3	4	6	4	8	5	30
1	Off	4	5	6	4	8	5	32
2	Off	4	5	6	4	10	5	34
3	Off	4	5	6	4	10	5	34
4	Off	3	4	6	4	8	5	30
5	Off	4	5	6	4	12	5	36
6	Off	4	5	6	4	12	5	36
7	Off	4	6	6	4	12	6	38
8	Off	3	4	6	4	8	5	30
9	Off	4	6	6	4	12	6	38
10	Off	4	6	6	6	12	6	40

SAMPLE 10-WEEK ADVANCED COMPETITOR TRAINING SCHEDULE: BUILDING FROM A 40-MILE-A-WEEK BASE TO 50 MILES

WEEKS	MON	TUES	WED	THUR	FRI	SAT	SUN	TOTAL
BASE	Off	4	6	6	6	12	6	40
1	Off	4	6	8	6	12	6	42
2	Off	4	8	8	6	12	6	44
3	Off	4	8	8	6	13	6	45
4	Off	4	6	6	6	12	6	40
5	Off	4	8	8	7	13	6	46
6	Off	4	8	8	7	13	6	46
7	Off	4	8	8	7	15	6	48
8	Off	4	6	6	6	12	6	40
9	Off	4	8	8	7	15	6	48
10	Off	5	8	8	8	15	6	50

WEEKLY MILEAGE GUIDE

RACE DISTANCE	NOVICE COMPETITOR	BASIC COMPETITOR	COMPETITOR	ADVANCED COMPETITOR
5K	10–20	15–25	25–35	30–50
10K	15–25	25–35	30–40	40–60
1/2 marathon	25–35	30–40	40–50	50–60

Note: These mileages should be averaged for 6–12 weeks prior to tapering for your race.

LONG-RUN MILEAGE GUIDE

RACE DISTANCE	NOVICE COMPETITOR	BASIC COMPETITOR	COMPETITOR	ADVANCED COMPETITOR
5K	3–6	5–8	6–10	6–12
10K	5–8	8–12	8–12	10–15
1/2 marathon	8–13	13–16	15–18	15–20

Note: Complete at least 3–4 of these long runs over the three months prior to your race.

TRAINING HEART RATE GUIDE

Training Heart Rate Range*

AGE	60 PERCENT	70 PERCENT	80 PERCENT	MAXIMUM
15–19	123–121	144–141	164–161	205–201
20–24	120–118	140–137	160–157	200–196
25–29	117–115	136–134	156–153	195–191
30–34	114–112	133–130	152–149	190–186
35–39	111–109	129–127	148–145	185–181
40–44	108–106	126–123	144–141	180–176
45–49	105–103	122–120	140–137	175–171
50–54	102–100	119–116	136–133	170–166
55–59	99–97	115–113	132–129	165–161
60–64	96–94	112–109	128–125	160–156
65–69	93–91	108–106	124–121	155–151
70–74	90–88	105–102	120–117	150–146
75–79	87–85	101–99	116–113	145–141

*Beats per minute as percentage of estimated maximum heart rate (220 minus age). Heart rate ranges listed correlate with age range listed. Interpolate to estimate your training range if you are between the age ranges.

Recommended Training Heart Rate Ranges

PERCENT OF MAXIMUM HR	RECOMMENDED FOR:
50–60	Easy walking and other moderate activity to introduce sedentary people to exercise, lose some weight, and promote health benefits.
60–70	Training range for easy recovery days and easy long training runs.
70–80	Recommended training range for maximum aerobic fitness.
80–90	Threshold between running aerobically and anaerobically; somewhere in this range you can't talk comfortably while running.
85–95	Hard training range and racing range.

Training Pace Guide

- **Brisk Pace** (10K + 1 min.) = approximately 80 percent of maximum heart rate; too fast for daily pace; do not run this pace on consecutive days or too frequently.

- **Base Pace** (10K + 1½ min.) = target for most runs; equals approximately 70 percent of maximum heart rate.

- **Easy Pace** (10K + 2 min.) = good for recovery days, equals approximately 60–70 percent of maximum heart rate.

10K RACE TIME (MINUTES:SECONDS)	10K RACE PACE	BRISK PACE (10K + 1 MIN)	BASE PACE (10K + 1½ MIN)	EASY PACE (10K + 2 MIN)
32:00	5:09	6:09	6:39	7:09
32:30	5:14	6:14	6:44	7:14
33:00	5:19	6:19	6:49	7:19
33:30	5:24	6:24	6:54	7:24
34:00	5:29	6:29	6:59	7:29
34:30	5:33	6:33	7:03	7:33
35:00	5:38	6:38	7:08	7:38
35:30	5:43	6:43	7:13	7:43
36:00	5:48	6:48	7:18	7:48
36:30	5:53	6:53	7:23	7:53
37:00	5:58	6:58	7:28	7:58
37:30	6:02	7:02	7:32	8:02
38:00	6:07	7:07	7:37	8:07
38:30	6:12	7:12	7:42	8:12
39:00	6:17	7:17	7:47	8:17

10K RACE TIME (MINUTES:SECONDS)	10K RACE PACE	BRISK PACE (10K + 1 MIN)	BASE PACE (10K + 1½ MIN)	EASY PACE (10K + 2 MIN)
39:30	6:22	7:22	7:52	8:22
40:00	6:27	7:27	7:57	8:27
40:30	6:31	7:31	8:01	8:31
41:00	6:36	7:36	8:06	8:36
41:30	6:41	7:41	8:11	8:41
42:00	6:46	7:46	8:16	8:46
42:30	6:51	7:51	8:21	8:51
43:00	6:56	7:56	8:26	8:56
43:30	7:00	8:00	8:30	9:00
44:00	7:05	8:05	8:35	9:05
44:30	7:10	8:10	8:40	9:10
45:00	7:15	8:15	8:45	9:15
45:30	7:20	8:20	8:50	9:20
46:00	7:25	8:25	8:55	9:25
46:30	7:29	8:29	8:59	9:29
47:00	7:34	8:34	9:04	9:34
47:30	7:39	8:39	9:09	9:39
48:00	7:44	8:44	9:14	9:44
48:30	7:49	8:49	9:19	9:49
49:00	7:54	8:54	9:24	9:54
49:30	7:58	8:58	9:28	9:58
50:00	8:03	9:03	9:33	10:03
50:30	8:08	9:08	9:38	10:08
51:00	8:13	9:13	9:43	10:13
51:30	8:18	9:18	9:48	10:18
52:00	8:23	9:23	9:53	10:23
52:30	8:27	9:27	9:57	10:27
53:00	8:32	9:32	10:02	10:32
53:30	8:37	9:37	10:07	10:37
54:00	8:42	9:42	10:12	10:42
54:30	8:46	9:46	10:16	10:46
55:00	8:51	9:51	10:21	10:51
55:30	8:56	9:56	10:26	10:56
56:00	9:01	10:01	10:31	11:01
56:30	9:06	10:06	10:36	11:06
57:00	9:10	10:10	10:40	11:10
57:30	9:15	10:15	10:45	11:15
58:00	9:20	10:20	10:50	11:20
58:30	9:25	10:25	10:55	11:25
59:00	9:30	10:30	11:00	11:30
59:30	9:35	10:35	11:05	11:35
60:00	9:40	10:40	11:10	11:40

Note: Runners slower than 60 minutes for the 10K often train close to race pace.

Speed-Training Guide

U se the following charts to help guide your speed training. One controlled speed workout per week (perhaps two) is recommended to improve race performance. At least one day before and after speed sessions should be easy days. These charts are a general overview. For more detailed information on speed training and training for specific race distances (from one mile to the marathon), consult *The Competitive Runner's Handbook.*

The charts refer to four levels of runners:

- Novice Competitor (NC): Races 5K–10K at slower than 9 minutes per mile.

- Basic Competitor (BC): Races 5K–10K at approximately 8–9 minutes per mile.

- Competitor (C): Races 5K–10K at approximately 7–8 minutes per mile.

- Advanced Competitor (AC): Races 5K–10K at faster than 7 minutes per mile.

The charts refer to three basic types of speed runs: intervals, hills, fast continuous runs. Warm up and cool down properly for each speed session. Interval runs consist of four variables: distance, number of repeats, pace, recovery time. The charts provide you with a range for the variables to allow you to adjust the difficulty of the workouts.

Five paces (based on your present race pace) are used in the speed-training charts:

- **Hard Pace** (H): 10K pace minus 30 seconds or faster (approximately 5K pace minus 20 seconds)

- **Fast Pace** (F): 10K pace minus 20 seconds (approximately 5K pace minus 10 seconds)

- **5K Pace** (5K): approximately 10K pace minus 10 seconds (5K pace)

- **Race Pace** (R): Goal pace for your race distance

- **Tempo Pace** (T): 10K pace plus 10 to 30 seconds (see Tempo on page 162)

INTERVAL-TRAINING GUIDE

DISTANCE	QUANTITY				PACE				RECOVERY (MINUTES)			
	NC	BC	C	AC	NC	BC	C	AC	NC	BC	C	AC
440s (quarters)	4–5	5–6	6–8	6–10	F-5K	H-5K	H-5K	H-5K	3–4	3	2–3	2–3
880s (halves)	3–5	5–6	6–8	6–8	F-R	F-R	F-5K	H-5K	4–5	3–4	3–4	2–3
Miles	2–3	3–4	3–4	4–5	5K-T	5K-T	F-R	F-R	4–5	4–5	3–5	3–4
1½–2 miles	1–2	2	2–3	2–4	5K-T	5K-T	5K-T	5K-T	4–6	4–6	4–5	4–5

HILL TRAINING GUIDE

Short hills	4–5	5–6	6–8	6–10	5K-R	F-R	F-R	F-R	Jog slowly downhill
Long hills	3–4	4–6	5–6	6–8	5K-R	5K-R	5K-R	5K-R	Jog slowly downhill

Note: Short hills should be 150–300 yards long and steep enough to challenge you (10–15% grade). Long hills should be 440–880 yards long and more moderate in steepness (5–8% grade).

Fartlek

After a 1- to 2-mile warmup, run 3 to 6 miles of "speed play" over varied terrain. Do surges at 10K race pace or faster for a variety of distances (50 yards to 1 mile) in a variety of combinations with a recovery period of approximately the same distance between them at training pace or slower. For variety, surge to landmarks (telephone pole, top of hill, etc.) or for a certain time (one minute, two minutes, etc.).

Tempo

After a 1- to 2-mile warmup, run 2 to 4 miles (or 15 to 30 minutes) at a brisk, steady pace that you can hold for the distance. For Novice and Basic Competitors, tempo pace is approximately 15 to 30 seconds per mile slower than 10K race pace, and training heart rate should be approximately 85 percent of maximum heart rate. For Competitors and Advanced Competitors, tempo pace is approximately 10 to 20 seconds per mile slower than 10K race pace and training heart rate should be slightly above approximately 85 percent of maximum heart rate. Tempo Intervals are an option: Run 10 to 20 seconds slower than 10K race pace for a quarter mile to two miles (or 90 seconds to 15 minutes). Keep the recovery period short (30 seconds to two minutes), and do a few more repeats than you would run for faster intervals for that distance.

Marathon Tempo Pace

After a 1- to 2-mile warmup, run 4 to 6 miles at marathon pace, or 6½ to 13 miles at marathon pace. A good option is to run a 10K to ½ marathon race at your marathon pace.

PART IV

The Marathon

Introduction to Marathon Training Schedules

The following marathon training schedules are from *The Runner's Handbook* and *The Competitive Runner's Handbook*. Consult these texts for detailed guidelines on training for and racing marathons. The schedules are part of the official training program for the New York City Marathon and the New York Road Runners Club (NYRRC) classes. Thousands of runners each year successfully complete marathons following these programs.

Please note these are *sample* schedules. Follow them exactly, as many runners around the world do, or adapt them to fit your needs. Use the daily mileage suggestions for guidance, as well as the following principles:

- Progressive increases in weekly mileage with a few plateaus and cutbacks

- Gradual increases in well-spaced long runs

- Off days and short runs for recovery to balance long runs and medium runs

- A gradual tapering of mileage and long runs over the final three weeks

Long runs are scheduled for Saturdays, but you may wish to change them to Sundays or other days. Carefully adjust your program to fit in a few races—adjustments could mean switching around long runs and running easy the day or days before and after the race.

These 16-week programs include a base level that you should hold for at least 3–4 weeks. Start with a comfortable mileage and long-run level, and increase your mileage and long runs following the sample schedules. Two schedules are included for the First-Time and Casual Marathoner (has completed marathons but with minimal training): one building from a 15-mile-a-week base for at least a month to 35 miles at the peak; and another starting at a 20-mile-a-week base and building to 40 miles a week. The second schedule is the preferred program. The Veteran Marathoner (Basic Competitor) schedule is recommended for experienced marathoners who wish to improve their times. The Advanced Marathoner (Competitor and Advanced Competitor) schedule is for runners who wish to train more seriously in an attempt to race a fast marathon. *The Competitive Runner's Handbook* includes several chapters with tips for improving your marathon times.

NOTE: The actual New York City Marathon training brochure is slightly different from the schedules here because it is adjusted to fit in official NYRRC races and long training runs.

MARATHONER'S MILEAGE AND LONG-RUN GUIDE

	WEEKLY MILEAGE	LENGTH OF LONG RUNS	LONG RUNS PER MONTH
First-Time/Casual	30–40	18–20	1–2
Veteran	40–50	18–22	2
Advanced	50–70	20–23	2–3

Mileage
Hold the recommended mileage levels for at least 6–8 weeks, then taper down over the last 2–3 weeks prior to race day.

Long Runs
First-Time and Casual Marathoners should complete at least three runs of 18–20 miles prior to the marathon; Veteran Marathoners should complete at least 4–5 runs of 18–22. At these levels do not attempt to run long every weekend, but rather every other weekend. Advanced Marathoners should run five or more runs of 20–23 miles. The last long run for all levels should be 2–3 weeks before the marathon.

SAMPLE 16-WEEK FIRST-TIME AND CASUAL MARATHONER TRAINING SCHEDULE: BUILDING FROM A 15-MILE-A-WEEK BASE FOR AT LEAST ONE MONTH

WEEKS TO GO	MON	TUES	WED	THUR	FRI	SAT	SUN	TOTAL
Base	Off	3	Off	3	Off	6	3	15
16	Off	3	Off	3	Off	8	3	17
15	Off	3	Off	4	Off	10	3	20
14	Off	3	Off	3	Off	13	3	22
13	Off	4	Off	4	Off	8	4	20
12	Off	3	Off	3	Off	15	3	24
11	Off	4	6	4	Off	10	3	27
10	Off	4	4	3	Off	16	3	30
9	Off	4	4	6	Off	12	4	30
8	Off	4	3	4	Off	18	3	32
7	Off	6	6	6	Off	12	5	35
6	Off	4	4	4	Off	20	3	35
5	Off	5	4	5	Off	12	4	30
4	Off	4	4	4	Off	20	3	35
3	Off	5	5	5	Off	15	3	33
2	Off	4	6	4	Off	6	5	25
1	Off	4	4	4	Off	2	26.2 marathon	14 + race

SAMPLE 16-WEEK FIRST-TIME AND CASUAL MARATHONER TRAINING SCHEDULE: BUILDING FROM A 20-MILE-A-WEEK BASE FOR AT LEAST ONE MONTH

WEEKS TO GO	MON	TUES	WED	THUR	FRI	SAT	SUN	TOTAL
Base	Off	3	4	4	Off	6	3	20
16	Off	3	4	4	Off	8	3	22
15	Off	4	4	4	Off	10	3	25
14	Off	4	4	3	Off	13	3	27
13	Off	5	4	5	Off	13	3	30
12	Off	4	5	5	Off	15	3	32
11	Off	6	6	6	Off	12	5	35
10	Off	6	4	4	Off	18	3	35
9	Off	6	6	6	Off	12	5	35
8	Off	5	6	6	Off	20	3	40
7	Off	5	4	5	Off	13	3	30
6	Off	5	6	6	Off	20	3	40
5	Off	6	6	6	Off	13	4	35
4	Off	5	6	6	Off	20	3	40
3	Off	6	6	5	Off	15	3	35
2	Off	5	6	5	Off	5	5	26
1	Off	4	4	4	Off	2	26.2 marathon	14 + race

SAMPLE 16-WEEK VETERAN MARATHONER TRAINING SCHEDULE: BUILDING FROM A 30-MILE-A-WEEK BASE FOR AT LEAST ONE MONTH

WEEKS TO GO	MON	TUES	WED	THUR	FRI	SAT	SUN	TOTAL
Base	Off	4	6	6	Off	10	4	30
16	Off	4	6	6	Off	12	4	32
15	Off	4	6	6	Off	15	4	35
14	Off	6	6	4	Off	18	3	37
13	Off	6	6	6	4	12	6	40
12	Off	6	6	6	Off	18	4	40
11	Off	6	6	6	4	12	6	40
10	Off	6	6	5	3	20	3	43
9	Off	6	6	6	Off	13	4	35
8	Off	5	6	6	4	20	4	45
7	Off	6	6	6	6	15	6	45
6	Off	5	6	6	4	20	4	45
5	Off	6	6	6	Off	13	4	35
4	Off	5	6	6	3	22	3	45
3	Off	6	6	6	4	15	3	40
2	Off	6	3	6	Off	10	5	30
1	Off	5	4	4	Off	3	26.2 marathon	16 + race

SAMPLE 16-WEEK ADVANCED MARATHONER TRAINING SCHEDULE: BUILDING FROM A 40-MILE-A-WEEK BASE FOR AT LEAST ONE MONTH

WEEKS TO GO	MON	TUES	WED	THUR	FRI	SAT	SUN	TOTAL
Base	Off	8	8	6	Off	12	6	40
16	Off	6	6	6	4	15	6	43
15	Off	8	8	6	4	13	6	45
14	Off	8	8	6	Off	18	5	45
13	Off	8	8	8	6	13	5	48
12	Off	6	8	6	6	20	4	50
11	Off	8	8	8	6	15	5	50
10	Off	8	8	8	6	20	5	55
9	Off	6	8	6	Off	15	5	40
8	Off	8	10	8	6	22	4	58
7	Off	8	10	8	6	15	8	55
6	Off	8	10	8	8	20	6	60
5	Off	10	8	10	8	16	8	60
4	Off	8	10	8	6	23	5	60
3	Off	8	8	8	6	15	5	50
2	Off	8	8	8	Off	10	6	40
1	Off	4	6	4	Off	4	26.2 marathon	18 + race

BOSTON MARATHON QUALIFYING STANDARDS

AGE GROUP	MEN	WOMEN
18–34	3 hrs 10 min	3 hrs 40 min
35–39	3 hrs 15 min	3 hrs 45 min
40–44	3 hrs 20 min	3 hrs 50 min
45–49	3 hrs 25 min	3 hrs 55 min
50–54	3 hrs 30 min	4 hrs 00 min
55–59	3 hrs 35 min	4 hrs 05 min
60–64	3 hrs 40 min	4 hrs 10 min
65–69	3 hrs 45 min	4 hrs 15 min
70–over	3 hrs 50 min	4 hrs 20 min

Back in 1973, a great motivator for my running was my desire to qualify for the Boston Marathon. Then, the time standard for all ages was three and a half hours (my standard now as a 50+ runner!). Reaching that goal in my early years as a road runner was very satisfying, and completing my first Boston was one of my biggest thrills in my running career. The Boston standards still serve as a challenge for many runners even if they don't run the event.

The abovementioned standards are the qualifying times for the 101st running of the Boston Marathon in April 1997. Qualifiers must be run on officially certified and sanctioned marathons in the year before the Boston event you wish to enter. For up-to-date information on qualifying procedures, write: Boston Athletic Association, Marathon Applications, P.O. Box 1997 (or the year you wish to compete), Hopkinton, MA 01748. Even if you don't run Boston, training to meet the qualifying standard is a good challenge for many runners.

Carbohydrate Loading Charts

Carbohydrate loading is a two-part system. Runners need to rest the body and stock the muscles with glycogen.

During carbohydrate loading, 70 percent of calories come from carbohydrates—preferably complex carbohydrates. With each ounce of stored glycogen you store three ounces of water. Be sure you are drinking plenty when carbo loading. You'll know you're properly loaded if you gain 2–4 pounds—mostly water weight.

CARBOHYDRATE LOADING AND MARATHON TAPER

DAYS TO GO	EXERCISE TIME	TRAINING DIET % CARBS
7	60–90 min	60
6	0–40 min	60
5	30–40 min	60
4	30–40 min	60
3	20–30 min	70
2	0–20 min	70
1	0–20 min	70
Race		

CARBOHYDRATE LOADING GUIDE BY BODY WEIGHT

BODY WEIGHT	CARBOHYDRATE	
POUNDS	CALORIES	GRAMS
110	1600–2000	400–500
115	1672–2090	418–522
120	1745–2181	436–545
125	1818–2272	454–568
130	1890–2363	472–590
135	1963–2454	490–613
140	2036–2545	509–636
145	2109–2636	527–659
150	2181–2727	545–681
155	2254–2818	563–704
160	2327–2909	581–727
165	2400–3000	600–750
170	2472–3090	618–772
175	2545–3181	636–795
180	2618–3272	654–818
185	2690–3363	672–840
190	2763–3454	690–863
195	2836–3545	709–886
200	2909–3636	727–909

CARBOHYDRATE VALUES FOR COMMON FOODS

SWEETS	CARBS	CALORIES
Fig Newtons (2)	20	110
Power Bar (1)	45	230
Yogurt—Dannon fruit	43	240
PopTart—blueberry (1)	35	210
Strawberry jam (1 Tbsp)	13	50
Maple syrup (2 Tbsp)	25	100
GU Vanilla (1 Pkg, 1.1 oz)	25	100
FRUIT		
Apple (1 med)	20	80
Orange (1 med)	20	80
Banana (1 med)	25	105
Raisins (1/4 cup)	30	120
Apricots, dried (8 halves)	30	120
Fruit Roll-Up (2)	24	100
VEGETABLES & GRAINS		
Corn on the cob (small ear)	48	210
Rice (1 cup)	21	100
Vegetable juice (V-8— 8 oz)	11	53
Carrots (12 "baby" or 1/2 cup)	6	25
Peas (1/2 cup)	21	95
BREADS		
Bagel (3.5 oz)	52	262
English muffin	26	135
Bread (2 slices)	23	135
Matzo (1 sheet)	28	115
Waffle, Eggo (1)	17	120
Bran muffin (1 large)	45	325
PASTA & STARCHES		
Spaghetti (1 cup)	44	216
Ramen noodles (1/2 pkg)	25	200
Potato (1 med, baked)	21	95
Yam (1 med)	48	210
Lentils, cooked (1 cup)	40	215
Baked beans (1 cup)	55	330

CARBOHYDRATE VALUES FOR COMMON FOODS

BEVERAGES	CARBS	CALORIES
Apricot nectar, 8 oz	35	140
Cranraspberry, 8 oz	36	145
Apple, 8 oz	30	120
Orange, 8 oz	25	110
Gatorade, 8 oz	10	40
Milk, 2%, 8 oz	13	110
Beer, 8 oz	10	150
Gatorload, 12 oz, 20% Glucose	70	280
Exceed High Carb, 12 oz, 24% Glucose	89	356

PART V

Reference Charts

Fuel and Hydration for Running

SUMMARY OF FUEL INTAKE FOR RUNNERS

DAILY

Low-fat, high-carbohydrate (60 percent of calories or more) diet.

BEFORE RUNNING

Eat a small high-carbohydrate meal two to three hours prior to running, or a liquid carbo meal or energy bar one to two hours prior. Drink 8 to 16 ounces of a sports drink 5 to 15 minutes prior to long runs or races.

DURING RUNNING

Drink 6 to 12 ounces of a sports drink every 15 to 20 minutes during long races. Banana pieces or energy gels also help. 30 to 60 grams of carbos per hour is recommended.

AFTER RUNNING

After long runs and races, consume 50 to 100 grams of carbos within 15 minutes, another 50 grams every two hours until you eat a regular meal.

SUMMARY OF FLUID INTAKE FOR RUNNERS

DAILY

Drink 3 to 4 quarts or more, at least half of it calorie-free water.

BEFORE RUNNING

Drink about 17 ounces of fluid two hours before running, particularly long runs in hot weather. Drink 8 to 16 ounces 5 to 15 minutes prior to running. A sports drink is recommended for races longer than one hour.

DURING RUNNING

Drink 6 to 12 ounces (6 to 12 large swallows) every 15 to 20 minutes. A sports drink is recommended for runs and races over an hour.

AFTER RUNNING

Drink at least 16 ounces. Drink 16 ounces for each pound of body weight loss from sweat. Continue drinking more for several hours after long runs on hot days. Drink until urine is clear or pale yellow.

AIR TEMPERATURE (°F)

APPARENT TEMPERATURE (WHAT IT FEELS LIKE)

RELATIVE HUMIDITY	70°	75°	80°	85°	90°	95°	100°	105°	110°	115°	120°
0%	64°	69°	73°	78°	83°	87°	91°	95°	99°	103°	107°
10%	65°	70°	75°	80°	85°	90°	95°	100°	105°	111°	116°
20%	66°	72°	77°	82°	87°	93°	99°	105°	112°	120°	130°
30%	67°	73°	78°	84°	90°	96°	104°	113°	123°	135°	148°
40%	68°	74°	79°	86°	93°	101°	110°	123°	137°	151°	
50%	69°	75°	81°	88°	96°	107°	120°	135°	150°		
60%	70°	76°	82°	90°	100°	114°	132°	149°			
70%	70°	77°	85°	93°	106°	124°	144°				
80%	71°	78°	86°	97°	113°	136°					
90%	71°	79°	88°	102°	122°						
100%	72°	80°	91°	108°							

APPARENT TEMPERATURE	HEAT STRESS RISK WITH PHYSICAL ACTIVITY AND/OR PROLONGED EXPOSURE
90°–105°	Heat cramps or heat exhaustion *possible*
105°–130°	Heat cramps or heat exhaustion *likely* Heatstroke *possible*
130°+	Heatstroke *highly likely*

ACTUAL THERMOMETER READING (°F)

EQUIVALENT TEMPERATURE (°F)

EST. WIND SPEED (MPH)	50	40	30	20	10	0	–10	–20	–30	–40	–50	–60
CALM	50	40	30	20	10	0	–10	–20	–30	–40	–50	–60
5	48	37	27	16	6	–5	–15	–26	–36	–47	–57	–68
10	40	28	16	4	–9	–24	–33	–46	–58	–70	–83	–95
15	36	22	9	–5	–18	–32	–45	–58	–72	–85	–99	–112
20	32	18	4	–10	–25	–39	–53	–67	–82	–96	–110	–124
25	30	16	0	–15	–29	–44	–59	–74	–88	–104	–118	–133
30	28	13	–2	–18	–33	–48	–63	–79	–94	–109	–125	–140

(Wind speeds greater than 40 mph have little additional effect.)	LITTLE DANGER (For properly clothed person) Maximum danger of false sense of security.	INCREASING DANGER Danger from freezing of ex- posed flesh.	GREAT DANGER

Questions to Ask When Injured

These are some of the questions we ask runners who become sick or injured. The goal is to discover the reason or reasons you developed your problem. Often more than one factor is involved. The basic question is, What have you done differently in your running or your daily routine that caused the problem? Use the following checklist to help you determine the cause of your problem or, better yet, to help prevent a problem from occurring:

1. Have you made any sudden changes in the quantity or quality of your runs: mileage, speed, hills, surface?

2. Are you taking time to recover from races and hard workouts?

3. Are your feet or legs structurally weak? (Your doctor may have to answer this for you.)

4. Do you have good flexibility?

5. Do you warm up and cool down properly for all runs?

6. Do you stretch properly?

7. Are your opposing muscles weak? (Abdominals, quadriceps, etc.)

8. Do you have any previous injuries that might make you vulnerable?

9. Did you return from an injury or illness too quickly?

10. Is your running form proper?

11. Have you changed running surfaces, or are you running on uneven or slanted terrain?

12. Has running on snow or ice changed your running pattern or form?

13. Are you undertrained for the races you are attempting?

14. Are you racing too frequently?

15. Have you changed running shoes, or are they worn down, or have you started wearing racing shoes?

16. Has your weight changed? Are you overweight or underweight?

17. Is your diet adequate for your training level?

18. Are you taking proper care of your feet?

19. Have you changed any daily habits, such as driving or sitting more?

20. Are you under additional stress?

21. Are you getting enough sleep?

22. Have you been doing other sports that might affect your running?

APPROXIMATE CALORIES EXPENDED PER 30-MINUTE RUN

WEIGHT (POUNDS)	PACE (MINUTES PER MILE)						
	12:00	11:00	10:00	9:00	8:00	7:00	6:00
100	200	215	230	262	300	350	400
110	208	225	242	276	315	362	418
120	216	233	250	284	325	370	432
130	234	252	270	305	350	410	468
140	255	273	292	320	380	450	510
150	272	293	315	356	408	476	544
160	294	317	340	378	440	500	588
170	310	338	365	410	465	540	620
180	328	354	380	431	490	574	656
190	344	372	400	452	518	602	688
200	360	392	425	473	540	630	720

Note: 3,500 calories expended equals one pound of weight loss.

FOR THE BEST IN PAPERBACKS, LOOK FOR THE

In every corner of the world, on every subject under the sun, Penguin represents quality and variety—the very best in publishing today.

For complete information about books available from Penguin—including Puffins, Penguin Classics, and Compass—and how to order them, write to us at the appropriate address below. Please note that for copyright reasons the selection of books varies from country to country.

In the United Kingdom: Please write to *Dept. EP, Penguin Books Ltd, Bath Road, Harmondsworth, West Drayton, Middlesex UB7 0DA.*

In the United States: Please write to *Penguin Putnam Inc., P.O. Box 12289 Dept. B, Newark, New Jersey 07101-5289* or call 1-800-788-6262.

In Canada: Please write to *Penguin Books Canada Ltd, 10 Alcorn Avenue, Suite 300, Toronto, Ontario M4V 3B2.*

In Australia: Please write to *Penguin Books Australia Ltd, P.O. Box 257, Ringwood, Victoria 3134.*

In New Zealand: Please write to *Penguin Books (NZ) Ltd, Private Bag 102902, North Shore Mail Centre, Auckland 10.*

In India: Please write to *Penguin Books India Pvt Ltd, 11 Panchsheel Shopping Centre, Panchsheel Park, New Delhi 110 017.*

In the Netherlands: Please write to *Penguin Books Netherlands bv, Postbus 3507, NL-1001 AH Amsterdam.*

In Germany: Please write to *Penguin Books Deutschland GmbH, Metzlerstrasse 26, 60594 Frankfurt am Main.*

In Spain: Please write to *Penguin Books S. A., Bravo Murillo 19, 1° B, 28015 Madrid.*

In Italy: Please write to *Penguin Italia s.r.l., Via Benedetto Croce 2, 20094 Corsico, Milano.*

In France: Please write to *Penguin France, Le Carré Wilson, 62 rue Benjamin Baillaud, 31500 Toulouse.*

In Japan: Please write to *Penguin Books Japan Ltd, Kaneko Building, 2-3-25 Koraku, Bunkyo-Ku, Tokyo 112.*

In South Africa: Please write to *Penguin Books South Africa (Pty) Ltd, Private Bag X14, Parkview, 2122 Johannesburg.*